ALWAYS HER DAUGHTER

ALWAYS HER DAUGHTER

BY

KELLI BRADLEY

SILVER TORCH PRESS

www.Thedevoteddaughter.com
Kelli@thedevoteddaughter.com

Printed in the United States of America.

Library of Congress Control Number: 2018965389
ISBN Print: 978-1-942707-97-4
ISBN eBook: 978-1-942707-98-1

Printed by Silver Torch Press
www.SilverTorchPress.com
JillSilverTorchPress@gmail.com

Dedication

In loving memory of my mom, Betty.

Thank you for teaching me grace under fire and the true meaning of love and courage.

Table of Contents

CHAPTER ONE
COMMUNICATION FIRST

By my mid-thirties, I was a driven career woman who was raised by parents with a foundation of integrity and independence. I was working, traveling, and well into building my life. My mom was living on her own, with manageable diabetes, and I was helping as needed. She lived in the house we grew up in which was huge so my efforts were focused on home maintenance, pet care, and being her daughter. I tried to warm her up to moving into a smaller place, but she didn't want my help. We talked for hours on end about the benefits of a one-level home. I wish she would've listened to me or that I had the support to know what to say and do before her health became a trial of terror.

She had health issues, but she was still driving, socializing, and running her own show; what I and everyone else in the family were accustomed to. Since I didn't educate myself on healthcare subjects until we direly needed help, she gradually grew sicker, and my back was always against the wall as I struggled to find solutions. At The Devoted Daughter (www.TheDevotedDaughter.com), we offer solutions that speak to long-term planning, not just when there is a health panic. In reality, you need to talk beforehand about what can be an inevitable family crisis with your parents' health. To hold back indicates an element of denial. I can speak to my own denial. You can retain your dignity and stature as a son or daughter while also empowered by knowledge.

In my family of origin, we were expected to toe the line even when we were little kids. You don't rip up your books or destroy property. After a ski trip, you need to wipe down your skis and put them away, and it did not matter how tired you were or how loudly you complained. You don't throw your coats on the floor. We grew up in a beautiful home, and we were expected to take care of what we had, be responsible, polite, and gracious. Both of my parents worked hard, and they wanted to offer us more opportunities than they had. Our parents made all the final decisions on important issues. There was no question they were the authority figures in our household. I had this value system embedded in how I behaved in the future as an adult, including stepping in and struggling with my parents when they were unable to make decisions about their own welfare. My mom wanted us all to get along, and my siblings and I have worked through difficult situations to make that happen, yet it may have overshadowed pre-emptive decision-making that could have had a better effect on my mom's health.

My brothers and I had a vision of our parents living healthy and full lives. After all, we grew up with four healthy, long-living grandparents. We spent a lot of time with them, taking trips and sleeping over at their houses. The assumption was that my parents would age the same and enjoy their grandchildren. As adults, we never thought about how things would be at our parents' ages. We were busy with our lives, exploring the world, and planning for our futures. Life has a way of course correcting.

I was utterly unprepared for what would occur with my mom's health over the next two decades. I was not equipped when I was thrown into the logistical and emotional aspects of continual and numerous health issues, as my mom declined in her fifties. I would take on the role of extreme caretaker, grasping to throw together information in stressful moments, wanting to implement the right action. I would be available at this pace; on call, for the next twenty years, until her death. I don't want the same scenario for you. You can have information delivered to you in an organized, orderly way. With The Devoted Daughters' Circles of Care, we have created in-depth categories containing content-specific information; all you need to know on your journey—technology, education, products and services, helpful people, and the information/data changes. Care is never linear, but it is overlapping. We have organized key guidance, tips, lists and direction in Circles of Care of how to care for your parent. The goal is to build a circle of care for people that say they don't have anyone. You do. You don't recognize what you have, so we start to understand where we can be empowered. With technology, we don't have to struggle or be alone in our decisions for care. You have the right to connect with others and gather information in a digestible way. I have been in the position as a daughter and caregiver of having no information hub.

When my mom's health started declining, our family was unprepared for debilitating illness. People wait too long to get help for their parents; I know I did. You can begin the process of understanding what needs to be communicated with your parent and extended family much earlier than you even think necessary. Educating yourself is a key element. Without knowledge, you're communicating blindly. My mom's health issues started when she was diagnosed with diabetes at age 47. She was in the middle of a divorce, dealing with my hard-to-handle dad, and her father had just died. At first, it was dealing with the day-to-day needs. My mom was independent and calling the shots, and I was busy with my obligations. At the beginning, she was able to manage her affairs. Her health was a concern, but it was not anything she could not handle. She was my mom, and she always took care of business, including herself.

I respected my mom in that role, and I was resistant to begin to parent my parent. She taught me right from wrong and how to be respectful of others. My mom hosted birthday parties, helped me decorate my room and pick out my school wardrobe from the Sears catalog. She was always at school attending PTA meetings and running the campfire girl meetings. My communication pattern with my mom was established at a young age. I was in denial that I would ever need to develop a different communication pattern with her that involved taking care of her and making the right decisions. She also was so young, so it wasn't natural how sick she became.

How we communicate with our parents as children is how we communicate with them as adults. I assumed this communication style with my mom would never change. Lifelong patterns are established at a young age and breaking those patterns later in life feels awkward and counter-intuitive when suddenly you are the one making final decisions about your parents' well-being. When did the person who picked me up from school every day start to need help paying her bills? My mom is the same, but now she is different. She can't do what she used to do. The vision of my mom needing this kind of help and support shook me to the core. I had to adjust my communication, instead of falling back on the old ways I expected her to have. I wish I had reached out to more people for support instead of being the lone ranger forging ahead. But the truth of the matter is, there were not any companies around like The Devoted Daughter. In-home care was in the initial stages of being established as an industry. Information was not available in the way that it can be now.

Despite my busy life at this time, my mom and I talked on the phone every day to check in. My brother, who was fourteen years younger, was still home. I used to run by my mom's house and check in with them. Life was as normal as it could be. When my mom's health started to decline more rapidly with complications from diabetes, she needed help managing her home. It was a large house and was filled with memories of raising her family.

I increased my time helping my mom with chores around the house. When I would call her on the phone, our conversations would be about her health, and I could hear her unravel. Pencils down, I have to go over there. Her legs and feet had neuropathy, which is extreme nerve pain. Nerve pain is one of the side effects of diabetes. At times she was unable to walk because of the illness. Today, there would have been scheduled in-home care helping to be sure her basic needs were being met so I could go to work and not be crazed. My thinking was unguided. I would wait until disaster struck, and then I would race over there to clean the sheets, the shower, and make sure all her hydration, nutrition, and medication needs were met. She was doing the best she could but if someone had been supporting her like a professional caregiver her condition may not have gotten to the crisis point.

If you have a parent that has been diagnosed with a chronic disease, the symptoms may be manageable at first. We never knew why, but with my mom, nerves in her gut may have been affected because she would have projectile diarrhea. It was horrible for her, and also for me who had to repeatedly clean it up. I was in the middle of so many facets of care. I would encourage you to learn more about your parents' specific diagnoses. How can you support them and what changes may be coming down the road? Have you tapped all the resources you can think of to get more information?

Luckily, it was not until my brother went to college that my mom started to be sick in bed for weeks on end. As she grew gradually sicker, her being all there mentally did not make it any easier for her to cope with all the medical issues. Our communication changed to where I had to assure her more than she was reassuring me like she did in my childhood. Here is where the People Category in The Devoted Daughter Circles of Care comes into play, which I talk about later in the book. Even if you don't have family to lend a hand, there are people you have not thought of so that all the burden doesn't fall on you.

Toward the end of my mom's life I opened an in-home care company. These experiences further solidified for me what sons and daughter need in the Circles of Care. I was asked in one of the assignments to help a woman named Annie to find care for her parents:

Annie's Story

"My parents were both living with dementia and wanted to remain at home. My dad was a retired physician and insisted that he did not need any help. I had two sisters and they had their own families. I was at my wit's end trying to help my folks and take care of my own family. The daily routine of getting my kids off to school, supporting my husband in his career, volunteering, and stopping by to check on mom and dad every day wore on me. I was desperate to find just the right person who would be able to reason with my parents, but since they were both living with dementia, that was not a realistic goal. I was relying on my communication skills and patterns from childhood. I wasn't able to focus on what was important, and instead organized the Tupperware as was taught to me by my mom. I organized the lids and put them all the same way, but in a few days they would all be a mess again because my mom has dementia and would go in there and play with the lids. I didn't see this at the time, but my communication with my mom would be as if a rational person, not someone living with dementia. I would say to my mom, 'You smell. You have got to get in the shower.'

"My mom would reply that she had taken a shower that morning and was insulted by the way I was speaking to her."

Unfortunately, Annie would accept her mom's answer and her mother wouldn't shower. She didn't have any coping skills.

Standing up to your parents is a challenging but pervasive problem when children become their parents' caregivers. Annie felt defeated; she could not convince her parents that she was trying to help, and she did not have the support of her siblings. They all wanted what was best, but each of them had their ideas of what should and should not be done. At The Devoted Daughter, we offer you icebreakers to start these conversations with siblings and family members before you are in too deep.

~~~~

I wasn't one to talk at the time. I could see it in other people, but not in my own behavior with my mom's sickness. I was plugging holes as needed and moving on as quickly as I could as her health declined. More discussion would have benefited the entire family because we were all going in different directions. Each one of us assumed that what we were doing was the right thing for my mom, but we did not talk about the individual contributions. We were still caught in the paradigm of her base wish—to just get along. We wasted a lot of time repeating chores that someone else had already done or making plans that had already been made. The Circles of Care encourages you and your family to evaluate individual roles and contributions. Taking the time to map out a strategy can improve everyone's experience during the caregiving process. The time we spent running in circles could have been quality time with my mom learning a new way of communicating and developing a relationship that would sustain us through hardships.

At the time, primary care providers were just coming into favor. You could directly call a specialist and make an appointment. Today, you need a primary care doctor to make referrals, and insurance rules are more complex with multiple networks,
~~~~

Medicare advantage programs, and the list goes on and on. Mom was making her appointments and attending them alone. We had no clue what was going on except what she shared with us. As she got sicker, it was much harder for her to advocate for herself. She would gradually forget to tell the physician everything he or she needed to know or to ask the right questions. It can be challenging to make the time to attend medical appointments, but getting the right information is vital. If you are unable to participate in the appointment, you might request to be conferenced in on the appointment or assign someone to be an advocate on behalf of your parents.

As a result of my mom continuing to run the show in her sickness, pieces of her life started to fall apart. Her healthcare needs were becoming too complicated for her to handle on her own. Then her frequent calls began. The phone would ring and I would hear a weak voice on the other end asking for help. I would jump in my car and head to her house to find my mom upstairs sick as a dog. Many days she had not gotten out of bed and was too weak even to make it to the bathroom. She had not taken her insulin or any other medication. It was a process to pull her out of this state, and many times it required a visit to the emergency room for IV fluids and medication intravenously administered. Her body was exhausted and challenged in so many ways.

I was blindsided. I was moving up the ladder in a large telecom company and had no notion of any obstacle. I had one objective: get in there and work your tail off if you want to be successful. There was a lot to handle already as a woman keeping her head above water in business. What were we doing, who was in charge? I did not have the tools to know to call a family meeting, which is precisely what I should have done.

At The Devoted Daughter, we show you how to execute immediate communication with your family. Family meetings are key to the success of your caregiving journey.

As soon as you have the idea that there is a health situation brewing for a parent, sit down and talk to your family about their wishes. Don't keep thinking it will go away or get better.

Parent cues to watch for:

- Falling behind on what should be a manageable task like following up on blood tests, paperwork, doctor's appointments
- Bills not paid on time
- Daily housework not getting done
- Mailbox is tipped over, but dad is usually really handy
- Garage and tools once neat and clean, are now disheveled
- Old food left in the refrigerator
- Parents no longer participating in activities they once enjoyed
- Personal hygiene habits have changed
- Loss of ability to plan their day or week

If you see any of these signs, then vital questions need to be answered:

- If something did happen, who would be there to help and in what capacity? Take some time to think about who does what in advance. For married couples, it is common to compensate for one another's weaknesses. For example, dad may drive, and mom does the cooking.
- If something happened to dad, who would drive? Mom quit driving years ago and she is dependent on dad to take her to appointments, shopping, etc. Would you or your siblings take on the role of driving your mom?

- Who would be able to step in immediately in case of emergency? Who lives nearby and who is available?
- Do you have a list of current contacts who would need to be notified?
- Do your parents have a legal or medical power of attorney?
- Do your parents have an advance directive or POLST?
- Can your parents maintain the same level of independence if one of them is disabled?
- Is there an emergency plan in place for help if needed? Have you thought about hiring professional help?
- Who will handle the day to day chores? Doing laundry, shopping, errands, mail, bill paying, and caring for the pets?

I have helped hundreds of families over the last ten years, and most of them struggled with knowing when the time is right to bring up planning the future for your parents. Many people are still living a full and vibrant life in their seventies. Your parents are doing well; you do not want to rock the boat, and conversely, if they are struggling it is not the right time to bring up what is already a controversial subject. Is it any of your business to insert yourself into their private matters? I would encourage you to break this down into baby steps. Who says you have to do it all at once?

Start by talking with the people who could be directly impacted by a change in status Once you have an idea, take it to mom and dad to inform them that we all agreed with this plan if changes are necessary for the future. Do not be caught off guard if your parents push back and say this is none of your business. They may tell you they need to talk about this in private or something to that effect. When you hear this kind of talk, you are experiencing a role reversal. You will need to trust that as an adult, you can see that mom and dad are struggling in a few areas and you can help. We were raised to take care of others, so now the others are your parents who taught you skills. Having this conversation can be harder than the conversation you had with your kids about the birds and the bees. It weighs heavy on your mind and your heart. Wanting to do the right thing can come at a price sometimes. Regardless of your upbringing, please give your parents who may be experiencing illness or normal aging some grace. It is important to consider what your mom and dad want. Can you honor that and be flexible?

People wait too long to ask for assistance on a deeper level that may not be apparent. Denial must be overcome, or it can get very out of hand. Trust me! When we assume things are fine or our parents want us to believe things are going well even if they are not, it is easier to deny that they now require more help. Many of the families I have worked with have the best intentions and believe that after a hospital stay dad is going to jump back on riding the lawn mower and haul yard debris to the dump. They want to be supportive and see how things go when they get home. Waiting to create a plan can be risky. It is hard to accept that as we age conditions change. Our parents cannot always do as they once could. That does not mean that your dad is no longer your dad. Meeting your parents or grandparents where they are instead of where you want them to be or where you think they should be can make all the difference in your relationship.

So, what do you do about family members who do not see eye to eye on the next steps when it comes to aging family members? These folks can make communication challenging.

I worked with a client whose kids got way too involved and then burned out. At the same time, they suddenly restricted what their mother could do. It is a snowball effect. Mary needed someone for real. If they had just stopped doing everything, we could have really seen what she needed.

Mary's Story

"I had been living independently for years after the death of my husband. One day at lunch I told my daughter, 'I think I am losing my mind.' My daughter attempted to calm me down, but I insisted that something was wrong. Over the next couple of months, my kids argued every day over what I should be doing and where I should be living. I had six kids and no one was on the same page. My future and my wishes had never been discussed. I was so sad that my kids were divided over my future. In the end, I gave up and decided to leave the family home to end the fighting. I decided on an assisted living facility not far from the family home. I figured at least I would still be living in the same community. I was accustomed to my grocery store; my hairdresser and my doctors were all close by."

~~~~

Conversely, when you do open up the dialogue, you will be surprised to learn who is willing to help. My mom had so many friends and was a very social person, but some of the most amazing gifts came from people whom I would have never expected. Completing your People Circle of Care will expand your options for care. I expand on the people who surprisingly stepped up to help me with my mom in later chapters. These people are often not who you would expect to step up. Figuring out who you can call in a pinch is also essential. Take a look at each person's skill-set, maybe one of your sisters is detailed oriented. She might be a great person to help with documentation or medication
~~~~

management. Don't be afraid to ask for the help you and your family need. People offer assistance willingly, but figuring out who is committed can be another story. If someone does offer, thank them and pencil them in to pick up your mom next week for a lunch date.

Changes to your parents are never linear. They can fluctuate, settle, and then take a turn for the worst or better. People can also mislabel their parents as having dementia. You can't just say that lightly. There could be a million reasons for a change in status. It could be hearing loss. It is so important to have your parent diagnosed and not just label them. Listen, learn, and do not make assumptions. Find out when mom or dad has had a complete medical workup. The Devoted Daughter's circle for personal information and data would house this information. Offer to help them make the appointment and go along. If they want privacy, offer to drive them to the office and learn as much as you can. When you participate as a health care advocate and the physicians know you are there to support your parents, they will be much more likely to help you gain a role in your parent's healthcare.

For each family, this is a different journey. Some people may require more help around the house after major surgery, and then the need for care levels off. If someone is accustomed to having a family member visit on a regular basis and for some reason that can't happen, look at some professional help to back up the support your family is already providing. As my mom's health continued to decline, I found myself spinning in the waiting room of a hospital knowing darn well that no one was going to provide my mom or me with the magic bullet to cure what ailed her. What I wanted was to help her have a new normal. Her circumstances would change once again. It was so hard to watch her lose her independence. At first, it was not making dinner for the family, not driving at night, and the need to hire extra help around the house. As time went on, feeling crappy and spending days in bed were more and more common. She also took longer to recover.

My lack of acknowledging that I would fall into the role of an almost-full-time caregiver prevented me from taking some critical pre-emptive actions that I can help you to understand. It was only years later that I looked back and realized I was providing intensive amounts of care and had lost sight on my own life, or the joy of my mom's and my relationship.

When I look back, I see how it slowly developed unbeknownst to me. First, I ran errands, supported my mom when she was not feeling well, and was an extra set of hands or eyes as she was losing her sight from diabetes. I did not think I should get some more help. Instead I was in the sadness of it all. *Why can't she just get better?* Or *She will get better soon if I do X, Y and Z.* My mom's goal was to remain at home. How could I make that happen (as a solo enterprise)?

There were fifty million people over the age of 65 in the United States alone in the year 2016. Our society is aging, and most of these people are living with two or more chronic health conditions like diabetes, heart disease, high blood pressure, etc. Take a look around the next time you are in the grocery store. There are a lot of seniors who use the grocery cart as a stability device. They don't want to use a walker because it is a symbol that tells people to be cautious. Your parent could be embarrassed by the signal the walker was sending to others. The scenario I just described may not apply to you now, but when the day comes that it pertains to your parent it will be a different story. You are not in it until you are in it, but you can start preparing now. Planning for the future is imperative. The Devoted Daughter offers you the tools and resources to start thinking about what is ahead for you and your family.

I lived through a horrendous physical downslide for my mom that spanned two decades. Through that whole time, I did not ask for the help I needed or have any tools for coping. She never would get well and grew continually worse. I also started an in-home care business because I knew so much about health care and assisting others through my experiences with her. The Devoted Daughter sprung from me deciding to leave in-home care and create a hybrid experience in one place for clients who needed the information that I and so many others desperately needed.

CHAPTER TWO

MAJOR CHANGES

I understand what you are experiencing. I have been there too. You have a hunch that your parent may be sicker than he or she is fessing up to but don't know what to do about it. Or you are struggling to push through and accept that rougher times may be ahead. My most significant transition mentally was accepting that I was now not just a daughter, but I was a caregiver. I always thought that was someone you hire to take care of your parents. I did not think of myself as a caregiver while doing just that for my mom. It was a natural progression as a daughter to take on the responsibility. Isn't this what every daughter would do for her family?

When my mom's diabetes was first diagnosed, none of us thought it was a big deal. My grandfather—her dad—had diabetes and it had not impacted his life in a significant way. She thought, *I will need to watch the progression, and everything will be ok.* Nothing could have been more false.

One move that we made, which was very smart, was to downsize her living situation. I wish I could take credit for making this happen, but she came to the conclusion herself. The house she lived in was our large childhood home that was surrounded by property that needed time and attention, not to mention the expense. I thought that she would be able to stay home if she had a smaller home to manage. She was entirely on board and ready for a new chapter in her life. My younger brother had moved out and she was making the decision to move for herself. I was so happy that she would have something to look forward to and a fresh start. Between her medical care and the expenses of maintaining a property of this size, it was time! She was sixty. The market was not high when we put the house on the market, but we could not afford to wait any longer. My mom was excited to move on, and she knew that her current home was too large and in need of ongoing repairs.

Once the decision to move was made and she found a new home, things seemed to be moving along nicely. Building a new house was a welcome distraction. It was also a relief not to have the financial pressure of maintaining a large home. On top of all the time spent on appointments, we spent over a year preparing the house for sale. My mom had lived in the house for over 30 years. Deciding what would stay and what would go was a painstaking process. She had all our childhood toys, clothing, and scrapbooks, and then all her personal possessions. Selling property and downsizing is not for the faint of heart, but having family support made the process more fun. My mom, Gram, and my mom's aunt sat around for hours preparing for the big garage sale. There were enough holiday decorations and paper napkins to entertain a cast of thousands. You would have thought this was a Neiman Marcus sale. Every last item was priced tagged and readied for the big day. They were her belongings, and she had pride for her home, the treasures she had collected over the years, and the memories associated with those items. What a fun weekend for all, with hope in the air that this move would change the trajectory of my mom's life.

I still find myself today looking at something that belonged to my mom and thinking about where it was in the house and what it meant to my mom. My great grandmother wrote notes on the personal possessions she wanted to hand down to someone in the family. My gram started doing the same thing, and it is so unique to have those notes and memories.

My mom found a lot in a neighborhood she thought was perfect. The home was on a hill with two stories and the master bedroom and bath upstairs. I didn't want to stand in her way when she purchased this house, but I had fears about her navigating the two floors. There was no way to modify the floor plan. It had everything she wanted. I took her to meet the builder and select the finishes. The decor was light and bright! She was so excited, and I wanted her to be happy. She had a little room for my gram and a place for my brother Chris when he came home from school. She also had a room that we fondly referred to as the junk room. It was an extra bedroom that was serving the purpose of a storage room. Doesn't everyone need a junk room?

She loved that house and enjoyed every minute she spent there, but her health continued to get worse. Diabetes had caused numerous side effects including neuropathy, loss of eyesight, and renal failure. She had so many doctors, I lost count. By the time I realized the severity of her healthcare needs, the train had already left the station. Her calendar was filled with medical appointments, tests, and calls to insurance companies that needed to be made. I had an indication she was going downhill even with the move. There were periods of time when she would be super sick and then she'd get better. She would do as much as she could, and then she would be on the living room couch passed out. She was pushing herself; I knew she wanted to carve out every opportunity to live her life. I wanted her to experience joy; why should I say you can't go on a trip or drive to the casino at the eleventh hour? It was her life, and she wanted to maintain her dignity and her relationships with her friends and family. My mom was not in a great financial situation. Her savings were limited, but she continued to shop and spend. We tried to have the conversation with her, but it was falling on deaf ears. As a family, we were able to come up with solutions and work out the funding, but if you don't have that option, you will want to start planning sooner rather than later. Reality has to set in much earlier than you think. At The Devoted Daughter, access the Tips on Money checklist which includes the importance of researching a power of attorney. How bills are going to get paid and the execution of the will can be a sticky wicket.

Just when I thought there could not be any more bad news, my mom was hit with a breast cancer diagnosis. It was decision time. What was the plan? What were the options? What did this diagnosis mean for her future? Since there were no care systems in place besides me and my brothers, we were more blindsided than you have to be not just by our level of involvement, but by the information we had to gather. The Devoted Daughter will be that place for you to go, offering information and resources to get you through to the next chapter of your life of caring for your parent.

I was struggling to figure out my own life. I was in the middle of divorce and establishing a new normal, but my mom's health had to be front and center. When is there ever a good time to find out your mom has cancer? The determination and drive my parents taught me kicked in like it was second nature. The minute my mom called with this devastating news, I said I would be right there. I told her that she was a fighter and that we would get through this. She would be as good as new before she knew it. I was not sure if any of this was true, but I knew that I would do my darndest to help her make that statement a reality. We got through the operation, but the surgeon messed up the reconstruction. I felt so awful for my mom; could she not catch one break with her health? When you see and hear someone you love experiencing any physical pain, it makes you question whether you are doing the right thing. I am supposed to be her advocate, her protector. Am I failing? Since she was an insulin-dependent diabetic, surgical procedures are risky. She beat the breast cancer and decided to live with the deformed breast tissue that was left behind. Often times, we forge ahead and tackle what we think are the most serious issues but we forget about the emotional toll this takes on the person living with the outcome of a botched surgery.

Many parents are in this situation. In my mom's case, her eyesight was getting worse with her health challenges. I don't know about you, but I can't imagine not being able to jump in the car and run to the store. The loss of freedom from giving up driving can be devastating. Having to rely on others for things can be very frustrating. A parent losing his or her independence can create social isolation.

Approximately 42.6 million adults over age 45 in the United States are estimated to be suffering from chronic loneliness, according to AARP's Loneliness Study in 2010. In addition, the most recent U.S. census data shows that more than a quarter of the population lives alone, more than half of the population is unmarried, and since the previous census, marriage rates and the number of children per household have declined.

So, how do we prevent elderly social isolation? Here are a few tips from The Devoted Daughter to offer your parents:

- Encourage your parents to get out and about. If transportation is not available, arrange for scheduled transportation. Many senior centers in local communities will transport seniors.
- Schedule visits around meals. It is often difficult to prepare food for one person and to enjoy a meal alone.
- For people who are housebound, meals on wheels provides hot meals and in-person delivery.

- Arrange for your parents to attend weekly events, book clubs, and other interactive forums are great to stimulate conversation.
- If you are noticing a change in cognition, don't jump to the conclusion that it is dementia. Have his or her hearing and vision been checked? It would not hurt to have a good physical from head to toe.

My mom insisted her vision was fine for driving, but we knew the diabetes was affecting her. One Christmas, my brother brought his girlfriend home; she is now his wife. He had not told her that my mom's vision was almost gone from diabetes. They arrived in the evening, and the first thing my mom said was, "Where is Lynne?" Lynne was standing right next to my brother, and my mom did not see her. It was clear she should not be driving. We asked her doctor to evaluate her vision, and she went to the DMV to speak to them about renewing her driver's license. I was dumbfounded when they renewed her license. You know your parents should not be driving, but they insist it is okay; they say things like, "I am only driving close to home during the daylight." What were they thinking? When you've exhausted all the reasoning, pleading, and begging, what are you to do about the parent that now insists on driving? You are now in the role of the scolding parent who tells the teenager they are not ready to drive! For many families, telling your parent he or she can no longer drive creates a massive bone of contention. I would suggest going back to his or her primary care physician to address the safety of your parents and others. If that fails, you may have to resort to taking the keys or even disabling the car. One of my clients who was living with dementia and did not have a current driver's license set up a test drive with a dealer. He convinced the dealer to drive the car to the assisted living facility where he was living. They let him take the car out for a test drive and he wrote the salesman a check for the down payment. It is scary to think this kind of thing could happen.

As I said earlier, not everyone may agree on what should happen next. Consider having conversations with your siblings separately from your parents. Hash things out in advance as much as possible so you can establish common ground. Check out The Devoted Daughter for examples you can use to start the conversation.

My mom continued to drive and got into an accident on her way home from dinner. The girl she hit was not hurt, but my mom fractured her left shoulder. It was a non-union fracture. These are very difficult to treat, but the physicians were hopeful that with physical therapy it would eventually heal. The fracture never healed, and it was not only painful, but she had limited use of her left arm. She had to use her right arm to lift her left arm above her head. The arm was no longer supported by the shoulder so it would hang down and pull on her body. I still get infuriated to this day to think about how we could have avoided this circumstance by not letting her drive and coming up with other ride share opportunities. There are so many more opportunities today for ride sharing. I remember driving around the hospital parking lot and jotting down phone numbers on the side of a car for transportation options. Planning ahead can make this so much easier, and reviewing your people in the circles of care will help shine a light on options you have not considered. The recovery was brutal and painful. My mom stayed with me for a couple of weeks so she was not alone. This was the first time she needed 24-hour care. At first, I was walking on eggshells trying to be quiet and keep her comfortable, but it was not long until she began trying to run the show. My phone started ringing off the hook. Cell phones were not like they are today, so all of her friends were calling my house to chat. I was trying to work from home, and honestly, it was driving me batty. My mom was eventually able to go home, but she now needed transportation to all her appointments, social engagements, errands, etc. We were fortunate that my mom had a lot of friends who were willing to drive and help out whenever possible. My brother David and I lived close by so we were able to jump in and help with transportation. It wasn't very organized; David and I were running in circles, so I highly recommend you make a driving calendar. The more organized and clear you are with who is doing what when, the better everyone will cope.

We were hardly out of the weeds though. One day, my mom was rushed to the emergency room with excruciating pain in her back. She was admitted to the hospital. She had suffered chronic back pain her whole life from a car accident that occurred when I was four.

As we waited for days for the orthopedic surgeon to get my mom in for surgery, she continued to experience pain that I could not imagine. My brother was in medical school at the time and came home to support my mom. The whole family was by her side. I had to leave the room when they moved her. I could not bear to hear or watch them put her through that kind of torture. I needed to walk away to stay strong. When they finally got her on the operating table, she was in trouble. Her bladder was full and she had some severe damage to her lower back. We were hoping the surgery would eliminate the pain and that she would still have full bladder function. The recovery would be a long, hard road.

My mom was never able to return to her new house on the hill. Can you imagine going into the hospital and never going back home again? I felt awful that she was facing so many health issues and now was losing her home. She loved that house and her belongings. She finally had a home where she could start fresh. The house was always decorated for the holidays and it was a gathering place for friends and family. My mom loved the sun, and one of her must-haves in the new house was a big deck where she could enjoy the sun and look down on her garden, especially the roses. I had no idea how I was going to break the news to her that she would not be able to go back home, but the stairs were a deal breaker. There was no way she would ever be able to navigate that home again.

We put the home on the market and again began the process of packing and staging the house. I gathered friends and family to carefully pack her belongings. It was just before Thanksgiving, and she had already decorated her kitchen table with a harvest motif. It was heartbreaking to have to take it all down. It took a couple weeks to get the house packed up. Once it was sold, we put most of her things in storage. I kept her most treasured possessions at my home. I packed them in small boxes and put them away carefully, thinking she would feel better knowing they were safe and accessible. I thought that she would enjoy using her dishware for holiday dinners even if we were not at her house.

My mom had so many treasures that had been passed down to her from her mom and grandmother. I have a glass cream and sugar set that belonged to my great-grandmother. When I was packing my mom's belongings, I found a note written in pencil on a torn piece of paper, tucked into the cream and sugar. It said, "Betty Ann, enjoy these and think of me often. Much love, Nanny." My gram was a note writer and wanted people to know the history of her belongings. Gram also spoke to members of the family and asked them if they wished to have specific items. When she first started asking us what we wanted, I have to admit I was a little put-off. I did not wish to have her belongings; I wanted her in my life! I have many of those notes today and treasure those memories. I did not know this at the time, but Gram would keep her memory alive by putting her stamp on things. She knew that one day we would look back on those conversations and thank her for sorting things out before she was gone. Just the other day, I found a cake plate with a lid. When I turned it over, there was a piece of scotch tape with Frieda (Gram's name) written on it. I felt Gram's presence at that moment. Although this is personal, it sheds light on how the spirit and the memory of those people you love can pop up.

My mom and Gram had planned a trip to Maui. They were so excited to get away and feel the warm sun and the sand between their toes. They had been looking forward to spending time relaxing and enjoying time away. My mom's neuropathy had gotten so bad, she could barely walk. Gram was taking care of everything, and on top of that, she was worried sick. My mom's future was uncertain, due to the increasingly challenging health issues. My gram talked about how it is not natural to have your child this sick. She wished on many occasions that she could trade places with my mom. Gram felt she had lived her life and she wanted more for my mom's life. I can't tell you how many times I have heard from both my mom and my gram saying that this entire situation is so unfair. My mom was angry with herself and her health. What I didn't see at the time was how isolated I was from the heaped-on responsibility as the caregiver.

Unfortunately, we were dealt this hand, but fortunately, as a family, we were committed to doing our best to make the situation for my mom better.

Through these major health issues, I didn't take care of my own social circle. My friends asked me to plan trips, dinners, all kinds of fun, but I was worried that if my mom was sick or needed something, I should be on call and available. Secondly, when I did have free time, I did not want to have any other obligations.

Tips from The Devoted Daughter to avoid caregiver isolation:

- Honor the time you have carved out to meet with friends. Arrange care for your parent in advance so you know you can take a break and relax.
- Have an accountability buddy who will not give up on you no matter how many times you say no to coffee, girl time, etc.
- Arrange for a professional paid commitment you feel obligated to attend. I hired a personal trainer to keep me on track.
- Stay engaged with your children and family during this time.
- Give back to others. I know this sounds counter-intuitive, but giving back to others fuels your soul and brings you joy.

Daughters and sons put out so much energy to care for their parents that at the end of the day they want to just be left alone. They lose their own selves. Conversationally, in a social situation, if people know you spend 99% of your time caring for someone else, they only ask about your parent's health, not you. When people would see me and ask, "How is your mom?" I appreciated that they were acknowledging what my family was going through, but I needed a social break. Let's talk about music, politics, and art.

Also, while I was in the throes of continual caregiving, my friends were enjoying their parents. Most of them had parents who had retired and they were able to spend time with their grandchildren and explore a new chapter in their lives. My mom was dealt a crappy hand, and I had the hardest time facing that fact. There are many ways to find support. If you are unable to find a group that is meeting locally, check out Facebook groups that might appeal to you. The Devoted Daughter has a private group for people to share information and get support. I was heartbroken watching my mom want to live her life and enjoy her friends and family, but struggle daily just to put one foot in front of the other. The undertaking was immense. I wanted to include her in everything we possibly could, and I would say to her, "You can be sick at home, or you can be sick with us." Not an excellent choice, but at least we were together.

While my mom had a tremendous support system, I remained the primary caregiver. My brothers, sister-in-laws, her mom, brother, aunts, uncles, cousins, nieces, and more friends than you can imagine were always in the mix. Arranging these people in the Circles of Care would have confirmed the massive team effort we had available at our fingertips. At times it was more than I could bear as a natural introvert, but people were well intending and wanted what was best for my mom. Everybody wanted information and updates. I would spend all this time in the hospital, and I would leave, and my gram would call and want to know more. It didn't exist then, but now there are online services like Caring Bridge to update people. One post to the site and all of your ailing parent's social structure is informed. It would have cut down the time I had to spend on the phone with all her acquaintances. I would've had more time to go home, work out, or go for a walk, especially when dealing with the Curious George People—people that weren't family or even close friends that felt entitled to the information.

As my mom's health continued to significantly decline, I did not look at the resources we had and ask for help. When you are in full steam ahead to survive and are also wrestling with all the natural emotions of your parent's pain or their losses, you adopt a mindset of I-am-going-to-do-it-myself. You assume only you can get it done right, and it will take less time. I also felt an obligation as her daughter to do it all, as she preferred that I was there; yet I wasn't there how I wished I could be, as a daughter and a loving companion. While caring for my mom could be a horrendous ordeal (and rewarding lots of other times), I learned all the ways I would have orchestrated her care differently. I didn't have the opportunity, but with The Devoted Daughter, I can offer you a comfortable and more simplistic approach to caring for your parents. We have all heard the saying, "It's the little things in life." No one can replace you as a daughter, but someone can go to the grocery store for you. That little act gave me the opportunity to do something for myself that day.

CHAPTER THREE

WHAT'S COMING NEXT?

I knew it was risky for my mom to live alone with all her pre-existing health conditions, but that is what she wanted. She would not have been happy any other way. It is scary when you know someone is vulnerable, but you are trying to honor and respect his or her independence. She didn't want to live in assisted living or have a caregiver there all the time, and I knew we would be facing some problems down the road because she was so insistent on remaining independent.

When my mom had to move from her new home due to her back issues, David and my mom went looking for an apartment. I remember the day they called me and said we found this great place that is close, has a pool, and you enter on the main floor. I was skeptical because it was all the way across town from me; at least a 45-minute drive. David said it would be better for mom. He felt he and Sarah could handle the night time and I could deal with the daytime. Oh boy, we had no idea what would lie ahead in the days and years to come. The calls to Sarah in the middle of the night started. My mom was incapacitated in some way and needed help to get back up, get cleaned up, or something urgent. She would apologize a million times over for waking them in the middle of the night, but she felt she had no other options. Thankfully, nurse Sarah was able to offer that much-needed help.

What do other people do that do not have this family support? In some cases, signs of aging go unnoticed until there is an urgent need. If no one is checking, an older adult can become vulnerable to health and safety issues. If you are not able to be there on a consistent basis, identify resources of people in the community who can provide support, such as senior centers, social workers from your primary care doctor, meals on wheels, or other volunteer organizations. You can also reach out to friends and neighbors so you have an extra set of eyes looking in on your parents. You can also check out The Devoted Daughter for a more comprehensive list of supports.

As my mom's health continued to decline, she could no longer engage in the activities she enjoyed and participate in a way that was stimulating and enjoyable. I realized it was time to employ some caregiving help, both hired and through friends. I discovered that accepting help from others could be more trouble than it was worth. Asking and allowing help will provide you with a needed break but don't say yes to everyone without knowing what is needed and giving them instructions. Getting in and out of the car or helping someone with a door can turn dreadful if not appropriately assisted. A caregiver taking my mom to dialysis was attempting to help my mom with the door. She allowed my mom to navigate the door and it hit her in the face and knocked her over. My mom was legally blind at the time. She had to be taken to the ER for stitches, one more ailment she did not need. Had the caregiver been instructed on how to hold the door, this incident could have been avoided. Never assume someone helping you with your parents knows them as you do. When someone offers help, don't be afraid to tell them what you need and hold them accountable.

Organize help in a way best suited for your parents, and then you are not managing the process all the time and having to do the task on your own in the long run. Be very specific with direction: it would be great if you could come by next Tuesday at 10:00 am and sit with my mom when she gets home from the hospital. Tell them you need the help, and be very appreciative of their offer.

As you deal with the physical changes in your parents, there are also cognitive changes that can occur, which can be frustrating and confusing. Who is this person that I have known my whole life in one way? You assume that you know who your parent is, but he or she may change in his or her older age, especially with dementia.

One of my clients, Clara, had been a well-respected English teacher for most of her professional career. Her son, Brad, hired us to provide care to his mom.

Brad's Story

"My mom loved to read, but she stopped reading when she was diagnosed with Alzheimer's disease in her early eighties. As the disease progressed, she started having more trouble following conversations. Her interest had shifted from reading novels to cutting coupons in the Sunday paper. One fall afternoon, I came over to visit, and found her sitting by the back door, clipping coupons. I was furious. I shouted, startling my mom.

"'Mother, what on earth are you doing?'

"She just looked at me with a blank expression, unsure how to respond. I was so disappointed that she was not doing something productive. She used to be this accomplished English teacher and now she has Alzheimer's disease, and nothing has ever been the same. The caregiver was also not using the time wisely."

Clara actually loved sitting by that little door with the breeze and the birds and the leaves blowing, but her son couldn't see that. He was short-sighted in not recognizing that Clara was in good hands because he was stuck in who his mom used to be, not who she was now.

~~~~

The Devoted Daughter can help you find a support community so you can pull yourself out of your disillusionment. Create a Facebook Group for other son- or daughter-caregivers with moms or dads who are sick at a young age, or that have an ailment specific to your senior. These people don't have to be your friends, but just sounding posts for your inner frustrations.

For my mom, the phone remained critical. She was always on the phone with friends when we were growing up and way after we moved out. My gram lived about 60 miles away in Salem, and she and my mom spoke several times a day; Gram always wanted to call my mom before she went to bed. That was a blessing and a curse. If my mom could not reach my gram, the alarm would sound and she was checking with family, neighbors, you name it, until she found her safe and sound. Most of the time my gram was snoozing soundly without her hearing aids, and none the wiser, the troops had been called. We commonly referred to the telephone as the Hotline. That crazy phone would ring off the hook. Everyone in the family was in the loop.

I inherited this habit because I did the same thing to my mom. I can't tell you how many times I called family, neighbors, friends, and even the non-emergency number for a welfare check.

Now, there is so much technology to use for your parents that reduces your phone time:

- The Echo Dot—You can talk to it, but it doesn't have a camera. I could've built my own network with my mom
~~~~

and had her easily call people if she fell. One time, I was not in town and tried to call her. She was not picking up. I called my sister in law, who went over there. She had fallen and was down all night. If technology had been in the home, she could've called out.

- Alexa Show (AI)—It's like the Dot but with a screen. You can stand and talk to that device and ask for healthy chicken recipes and it can also call people.

All these programs have music to build your own playlist. That is a nice task for grandchildren to do for their grandparent, or let's make a library of old movies or download interesting podcasts they can listen to.

To improve care and keep people out of the emergency rooms, technology is becoming more a part of our medical system. We are already seeing the new technologies, such as wearables, for tracking and collecting data. Caregivers are also using sensors in the home to track movements. If someone has not moved from the chair for hours or a habit has changed, an alert can be set to check on your older adult. I am not suggesting personalized care replaced by technology but it does reduce the anxiety of not knowing what is going on in the home.

I wished the Alexa technology had been available to my mom. She was blind from diabetes, and using artificial intelligence technology would have made many things so much easier for her. She used a talking clock, but that meant she had to have it nearby so she could push the button. With Alexa, you can ask what time it is. There are now assisted living centers incorporating wellness centers on-site to take vital signs and a video conference with a medical professional to eliminate some face-to-face doctor's appointments. Video calls can be beneficial and reduce the stress and anxiety of going to doctor's offices. It took hours to help my mom get ready, get in the car, and into the appointment. Not to mention it was hard on her. She did not feel well and using the little bit of energy she had to go to a doctor's appointment was discouraging. At one point, I counted all the physicians my mom had seen, and it was over 40 providers.

As the intensity of my mom's care needs was increasing, I felt an all-consuming pressure. I was always waiting for the other shoe to drop; what was coming next? She was in a tremendous amount of pain, and recent back surgery had not resolved the issue. We were on a first-name basis with the staff in the emergency room. I was frustrated I could not help my mom. Her health was spiraling out of control. I questioned the validity of every test and diagnosis. Trust someone to make the best decision who doesn't even know my mom? Sitting in the emergency room waiting for test results is painstaking. One evening, the physician gave us lab results. I called my brother Chris and read him the results. I asked him if there were any other questions I should ask. He instructed me, and I went back to the ER doc and told him. The doctor thought it was a good plan then looked at me and said, "What do you do?" I laughed and told him that I was cheating. These were not my original thoughts, but you have to do what you have to do to be thorough.

I am a do-er. Sitting around is counter-intuitive to my nature. Given a choice to clean the house or sit and chat, I prefer to clean. My mom and I spent endless hours of time in waiting rooms, driving to appointments and sitting in hospital rooms. I was very antsy and always living in the future to-do list. If I could turn back time, I would have cherished those moments with her and found the joy that on the surface I wasn't able to feel. I was always consumed with the task at hand. I missed opportunities for intimacy with my mom in these days, months, and years. I let others take the lead on striking up conversations and spending time just visiting. Keeping busy distracts you from what is happening. I kept thinking if we push forward, we can fix this.

My brother, David, was on the same page in many respects. He was always encouraging my mom to walk and eat. Maybe that would fix everything. I think we both suffered, knowing that underneath it all there was a space we could not fill. We were avoiding the pain of intimacy with our ailing mom by always doing and telling ourselves our actions were necessary to keep her alive. I know now that many of these actions we took were for us and not for my mom. Our hearts were always in the right place and my mom was such a trooper. She would do anything we asked that was within her power. She knew we were fighting for her and she so wanted to get better.

I founded The Devoted Daughter to support families just like my family, or more specifically, the sons and daughters who felt out of gas and not able to see the value of having a relationship with his or her parent despite what needs to get done.

We did everything we could imagine to advocate, care for, and support my mom, but I was so tired at the end of the day, when she would say, "Honey, can you stay a little longer?" I would feel guilt about desperately wanting to go home and recharge.

I wish that I'd had a resource like The Devoted Daughter to access information when I would think I was losing my mind. Who should I call?

I have been there!

With so much doing, we needed to be reminded to tap into our own feelings and acknowledging moments of grief. After all, she was slipping away right before our eyes.

There were times I would concede to stay longer, even though I just wanted to go home and snuggle with my dog, Rocky. There were also days when I just needed to leave. My mom did not realize the time commitment. Many days, I was there from early in the morning to early evening, and even when

I went home, she was always on my mind. I would get in my car and call my gram to give her the daily update.

Honestly, when Chris would come home from medical school, I would get the heck out of town. I needed a break, free from worry. There wasn't as much worry, yet that would come down the pike in my mom's health as the years passed. My mom was dependent on me for many reasons, and as time went on, I created a sense of responsibility every day and didn't ask for enough help. I was not convinced that people would follow through, so I developed a position of command central. I remember one year when Chris came home for Christmas break, and my mom had already lost her vision from diabetes. Chris and my mom would make goodies for Christmas day to be shared with the family. My mom was looking for something in the frig and could not see anything, so she asked Chris to call me. He did, and when my mom asked where the mustard was Chris said, "Mom I am right here; I can see. You don't need to call Kelli." At the time, we did not have cell phones with a camera, so before I would leave for the day, I would memorize where everything was in the frig so if my mom called me, I would be able to tell her where to find what she was looking for.

Putting the systems in place that allow you to delegate are key. There are nuances to care that can't necessarily fit your skill set. Be honest with yourself and know how much—and what—you can do for your ailing parent's situation. As a family, if you agree to a task like taking mom to the doctor, do what you say you will do. You need to fulfill your end of the bargain because when you don't, you are letting down someone else in your family, but ultimately, you are letting down the parent you are all working to take care of. It is such a letdown when a primary caretaker is already at his or her wit's end (and that was often me), and then someone lets him or her down. There are enough disappointments when you are helping someone with a complex medical condition. I always felt like the little things should be able to go smoothly. How hard is it to make some soup and drop it off? If support is offered but the person never follows through, don't beat your head against the wall and keep asking that same person for help. Understanding who your family members interact with is vital when building the support needed. Do not disqualify someone before you speak to them. What is the worst thing that could happen? They say no, and you move on.

Here are some Devoted Daughter Tips to make delegation a smooth transition:

1. Don't delegate medications to family members who are terrible at organization!

   There are so many rules around meditations. You need to delegate to someone detail-oriented who can be quiet and do the organization of the pills. I would go back afterwards to double count and check. I would make sure there were syringes with the right amount of insulin, see that next week I will run out of that med and get it filled.

   Seniors also can spill their pills. The medication boxes that are made of plastic can be hard to open and close. When opening, they can snap sending the pills flying in every direction. I can't tell you how many times I would go over to check on my mom and find pills under the chair, on the kitchen floor, and in the furniture. We always had a list of medications next to the box. You should know the type of medication, the dosage, the time it should be taken, and how it should be taken. When in doubt, you can always refer back to the list as your guide. Also, pharmaceuticals can change the color or shape of the pills and that can be very confusing to people. Your pharmacist can be a great free resource. During my career as a home care operator, I was faced with helping people organize their medication. A sweet older couple who had been married since the thirties was trying to make sense of new medication orders. I was not familiar with them, so I loaded up all the medications and paperwork and took them to their local pharmacist. They had no kids. He had a heart attack and the hospital sent him home in a medical transportation van. He got home and showed me all the paperwork, new orders for medications, and orders to stop taking other medications. This can be so confusing for people and they need help.

2. Make a primary calendar for your support system.

    There will be some people who can do more than others can, but figure out how to plug the holes. Make sure you engage and thank people for their time and effort. You might be thinking this is one more task that has been added to your plate, but a simple phone call or a thank you will go a long way. Identify the critical items like medication and transportation. Applying this advice is not limited to your parents. My sister in law was going in for surgery and I was taking care of her kids. I told her to write down everything she did for her kids every day, and I know it is a lot more than you are even thinking about. She said, "You are right, you forget how much you get done," and she won't be available for two weeks. What happens around the house that needs to be done? For elderly people, you don't need to take over if they are able.

3. The most unexpected people show up to help you in a pinch.

    I was surprised by people who I would never have expected to be there. The woman who did my mom's hair would have been there day or night to do anything we asked. My mom had a housecleaner who came every week and helped her with many things. This woman worked another full-time job but was there for my mom. It was important that things stayed clean not only for personal preference but for health and safety reasons. My mom was also there for her and her son. She was a single mom, and I think the relationship worked for both parties. It is incredible the gifts that can come into your life when you give up judgment.

4. Remember when I explained you may not know who your parent is anymore? Don't make judgments on caregivers based what you believed your parents' biases still are.

   I once had a client whose daughter assumed she was the same with dementia than before, and would never like a caregiver who was touchy feely.

Mrs. Brown's Daughter's Story

"My mom was living with dementia and vision and hearing loss. I was adamant about what should be done for her care. The situation was complicated because her case involved a third-party professional guardian, since my sister and I were unable to agree on what would be in the best interest of mother. The guardian was responsible for filtering the communication between family members and making the final decisions on all matters concerning mother's care and finances. I believed that my mom was not a touchy-feely person and that if the caregiver even got close to her that she would most likely accuse them of sexual harassment. I also believed the house needed to remain as it was. Kelli tried to gently point to the medications that were all over the kitchen counters and coffee table, suggesting we should come up with a safe way to organize and administer her medication. I felt resistance, even though I knew the medication should be organized. No one knew my mother like I did.

"Over time, Kelli and her caregivers realized that Mrs. Brown (my mom) welcomed touching. She was still Mrs. Brown, but she was different now. Dementia and loss of vision and hearing had altered the way she could take in new information. Her sensory input was limited, but she could still feel, and she could still smell. She loved jewelry. Whenever Kelli went over to visit, and she would thank her for coming, and sit down right her next to her. *Who was this woman?* I thought. *Definitely not the mom I grew up with!* She would always put her withered hand on Kelli's lap and reach up to her neck to touch her jewelry. The love of bobbles was something they had in common. I never wore any jewelry. My mom was not afraid of touching, and in fact, she was welcoming this more intimate interaction. By touching Kelli's jewelry, she pictured in her mind what it must look like. The caregivers also discovered that baking brought back a lot of fond memories for her. The house was filled with the aroma of freshly baked cookies. Had I taken the time to learn more about who my mom was today, I could have been more directive in who she would spend time with and enjoy."

~~~~

There are times when an outside person will have more success working with your mom than a family member will. Ironically, I did not see this when I was caring for my mom. I was all in to help with whatever she needed. It would have been helpful to introduce an outside person earlier on and start to build more support for my mom and the family. There is no history with an outsider and they are starting fresh. It can be hurtful to see a complete stranger helping your mom, and when you arrive, you
~~~~

get the cold shoulder from your own mom. Try to remember that for the most part, this kind of behavior may be disease-related, or chalk it up to the fact that we sometimes hurt the people we love the most because we know we will be forgiven.

I could have helped myself more as my mom had a pretty full social life. One day, I couldn't find her; I even sent the police as a welfare check, only to discover she and her friend, Joyce, were buzzing around in the Cadillac, going to the casino to get margaritas. She said "I felt good today, so I decided to go." I was like, "You don't get to take off," but I was not only questioning her desire for joy; I was losing out on my life by micromanaging. I was sitting around worrying about her on a beautiful Saturday afternoon. When I was done at the end of the day with all the little parts of her care or unnecessary worry, add in my work and life; I was spent and could only handle the Hallmark Channel.

CHAPTER FOUR

YOU CAN'T DO IT ALONE

I spent a tremendous amount of time with my mom in and out of hospitals, nursing homes, and assisted living. Because of that, I had the confidence to question the recommendations. I know this is not true for every family, but don't be afraid to advocate for your family members and ask for clarification so you fully understand why a recommendation is being made, especially when dealing with seniors.

My gram was living in her own home until she was 98. For two years, she would drive by or have someone go with her to check out the progress of a new independent living facility a stone's throw from her home. The sales agent must have met with her at least fifteen times during those two years. When push came to shove, she did not want to move there, or anywhere, for that matter. She eventually had to be moved, but it was not without a fight. She had heart problems, and her vision was not as good as it once was. Macular degeneration was setting in, limiting her ability to see. Gram's house had been the gathering place for the entire family for years. She lived on the river and enjoyed working in her yard and entertaining anyone who popped by. There was always someone from the neighborhood, a family member, or friend paying a visit. Uncle Bob stayed with her weekly, and I had her come to my house to visit for a couple weeks. Her back and legs were giving her problems, and we were afraid that she might fall on her stairs. There was not a bathroom or bedroom on the main floor in her home, so we all knew staying home was not a long-term solution.

The idea of moving was great when it was just a fleeting thought, but when reality set in, that was a whole new set of circumstances. We talked about all of the options; maybe she should move closer to me so I could see her every day. The decision of where to live was not about what was best for me but what she wanted. Staying in a location where she already had a support system made the most sense. Little things like her hairdresser, the pharmacist, doctors, friends, and just the familiarity of a place she had lived her entire life were most important. If she was going to get through this move, it was going to take the whole community. We got her settled into the independent living home, but it would never compare to living in her house. How could we ever expect it would? But it was the best solution.

One day, we were walking down the hall, and she said, "Kelli, this is just fine if you like this kind of living." She went on to say that she did not appreciate being with a bunch of old people. I gently reminded her that she was the oldest resident in the facility. Telling her that she was the queen of the castle did not change her mind about living in a facility. I can't imagine being that powerless against my own will and having my poor health due to aging dictate my lifestyle, but that is what our aging parents are facing.

Most people fall in one of two categories; they are either productive people or more social people. My gram was definitely in the productive class. She was the happiest fussing around the house, doing laundry, cleaning, cooking, and working in the yard. At the end of each day, she felt better about checking things off her list and living in a senior community did not offer her any of the daily task work she was accustomed to accomplishing.

According to the U.S. Department of Health and Human Services, around 70% of adults over the age of 65 will need long-term care at some point, but when asked, 90% of seniors want to stay home. So how do you help your parents plan for the future? The planning process doesn't come with a roadmap, and there are so many options to choose from. What may be ideal for your parents today may not be realistic tomorrow, so now what? Below, I have broken down some of the most common senior housing options so you can get a grasp on what is best for your family.

Adult day care

Daycare is an excellent option for those who need more socialization and a limited amount of medical intervention. You also get a break from your parent following you around all day asking you what time it is. For seniors living alone or those living with a family member, they may find themselves spending a lot of time alone with a lot of idle time on their hands. If your parent is no longer driving, their daily obligations are more difficult to meet and their social life is stinted. Leaving mom or dad at home while you go to work is worrisome.

The options for daycare continue to expand. For example, there are now daycare facilities that work with young children and adults; disease-specific options for dementia and Parkinson's patients are also available. Spend some time doing your homework and visiting different facilities. The Devoted Daughter can show you more specific lists of what to look for in top-quality day-care facilities and the questions to ask. The cost and the environment should be conducive to your mom's or dad's needs. Considerations should also be made as to where the facility is located. Most daycare operators have specific drop-off and pick up times for various programs, but some also offer to pick up mom or dad from home.

Don't pigeonhole yourself into thinking you need to select just one of these options. My client, Carol, and her husband, Dick, were struggling with how to balance their lives with Carol's Alzheimer's diagnosis. They were on a limited budget, and in-home care was not affordable on a daily basis. Carol loved spending time with her grandchildren, so I suggested a combination of adult day care and in-home care to meet Carol's socialization needs and budget. The daycare Carol attended had pre-school children who also participated. The interaction between the seniors and the young kids was fantastic. Their innate curiosity brought out the best in one another.

In-home care

In-home care is an excellent option for people who want to continue living in their own home. An agency will provide non-medical caregivers who will come to your parent's home to help them with basic tasks such as bathing, dressing, meal preparation, medication management, basic housekeeping, laundry, transportation, grocery shopping, or socialization.

Don't let the term non-medical throw you off. Each state has its laws, but in many cases, in-home care can offer a higher level of care. Keep in mind that you can use services that complement one another to provide the best experience for your family. As an example, home health could be supporting your mom when she gets home from the hospital after surgery, but home health only provides support on a limited basis. A home health nurse evaluates the patient and a recommendation for services is submitted for approval. Home health offers services like medication management, physical therapy, occupational therapy, and even bath aid assistance. To qualify for these services, the individual must require support in a home environment. There is more detailed information at The Devoted Daughter to help you differentiate between in-home care and home health. Home health visits are scheduled based on the availability of the provider. Don't assume that home health will stay with your mom for a couple of hours while you run errands. Working with an in-home care company can provide you with the flexibility you need while maintaining health and safety for mom and dad. In this case, in-home care and home health work together to meet the client's needs. In-home care can be engaged regardless of where your parents live. It is an excellent option for short- or long-term support.

I worked hand in hand with many home healthcare companies during my time as an in-home care owner/operator. My client, Ron, had been released from the hospital after having cardiac issues and hip replacement surgery.

Ron's Story

"I was confident in my ability to manage my affairs independently, but the hospital discharge planner saw things differently. The recommendation to go home was based on having round the clock care and the supervision of home health. I know I am a tough old bird and did not want to go home without fighting for my independence. I was in a setting with support so it was easy to forget that it might not be as simple to do things alone as one would think. That said, I was sure I could manage my medication, prepare meals, and shower by myself. That was not the case, so I needed Kelli and her staff to make me as comfortable as possible. It is invasive and downright strange to have someone in your home rumbling around to care for you, but that is what needed to happen."

Home health worked with Ron's doctors to get his medication and assistive devices ordered. We worked with home health and Ron's family to line out a plan of care to support Ron at home. It was not perfect, but it did the job in getting him back on his feet and keeping him safe at home. It also gave my team a medical resource around the clock in case of emergency.

~~~~

At The Devoted Daughter, I have a video that goes into even more detail on home health versus in-home care.

During my time as an in-home care owner/operator, we served over a thousand families. For each of those families, the supports were similar but different in many ways. You are working with individuals, and everyone is different. I would recommend you first meet in person to understand better what the agency has to offer. We have some great tips at The Devoted Daughter to walk you through this process.

Home health

Home health provides care in the patient's home with the supervision of a medical doctor. One of the main benefits of home health is that allows the patient to return to a home setting while still receiving a scheduled amount of skilled care. The patient cannot typically leave to get treatment, so the treatment comes to the home. For example, many people require physical therapy when recovering from an illness or injury. Rather than the patient leaving home, the physical therapist will visit the patient in the home and provide treatment in a home setting.

The home health team relies on the patient being at home. They will typically call to schedule a visit the same day. Home health visits are supervised by an RN. The RN will determine how long and how often services need to be provided, until the patient is no longer improving or benefiting from the services offered.

Here are a few more facts on home health:
~~~~

- The service is prescribed by a doctor in order for it to be covered by most insurance policies.
- 24-hour on-call staff is available.
- Be sure to ask about home health before leaving a hospital or skilled nursing facility or scheduled surgery.
- There are restrictions on when home health can be prescribed so arranging care in advance is critical.

Independent living

You need to move your parent out of the home. Downsizing is happening for many people, from the home they have raised their kids in to a two- or three-bedroom apartment. Many people become weary of taking care of a home and all the responsibilities that come along with that. Independent living is for the parent who is ready to take off in a moment's notice and enjoy the freedom of retirement. They are not typically sick or needing medical care on a regular basis. The independent community typically offers meals, housekeeping, laundry, social events, on-site amenities like a gym or fitness studio, and much more for the active retiree.

In some cases, you can even travel to locations under the same ownership. For example, someone living in Oregon could fly south for the winter, booking an extended stay at a sister property. These types of living arrangements are not conducive to those who need more help with things like dressing, bathing, and hands-on care. If your parents are living this lifestyle and one of them falls ill, you can supplement the living situation with outside help from an in-home care or home health agency.

Assisted living

If your parent has health challenges but does not need constant care, assisted living may be an option for you. Your loved one will have his or her own apartment but can attend shared meals and activities with other residents if he or she desires.

Assisted living centers vary significantly, as each state has different licensing and regulation requirements. Even if you're looking at facilities in the same state, it's important you spend time researching and touring each center. Make sure you understand the staffing levels. Services offered and delivering on those promises can be two different things.

In general, most centers will assist with the following:

- Activities of daily living (ADL'S) such as bathing, toileting, dressing, eating, shopping, etc.
- Regular meals
- Housekeeping and laundry
- Transportation
- Social activities
- Exercise programs

Costs will vary depending on the size of the apartment, services, area, etc. It's important to ask each community about the price and what services are included, if there is a basic rate charge. Some will consist of all essential services with additional costs or points for special needs, but most will tack on entrance fees, deposits, and housekeeping fees.

My friend, Sue, called me the other day asking what I thought about her mom going in assisted living. As we started to dig deeper into the conversation, it was clear to me that her mom thought she would have people helping her around the clock at her beck and call. Let me tell you this is not the case. So many times, I have walked through these huge buildings whose occupancy is filled, thinking to myself, there are a lot of lonely faces in these halls. Don't assume that just because there are a lot of people living someplace that your mom will be taken care of all the time. It struck me as I was talking with Sue that her mom's expectations were not realistic. She wanted someone to check on her every two hours around the clock. These facilities are not staffed for hourly oversight of their residents. If they can provide oversight to residents, there would be a charge or what they call points (dollars) associated with this service. My advice is to take your time visiting different communities at different times of day. Depending on what your parents are looking for, they might find that one facility suits them much better than another.

Memory care

Memory care is specifically for seniors living with dementia; the most common form is known as Alzheimer's disease. Memory care is a locked unit designed to meet the needs of the residents. Many times, the rooms are shared rooms, but private rooms are available. The cost is significantly higher, as the level of care required is also higher. Some assisted living communities offer this option as an alternative to assisted living. I would recommend touring all the possibilities when visiting communities offering a continuum of care.

Memory care units are often located on a campus that offers a continuum of care. For example, there will be a section of the campus for independent living, another for assisted living, memory care, and skilled care. There are even high-rise buildings that offer multiple levels of care. These are good options for someone who needs more care short-term and can then return to their apartment in another section of the campus. Multiple levels of care also benefit couples who need different support systems. Dad has dementia and needs memory care help, but mom is okay living in independent living. Mom can drop in on dad for visits, but she is not responsible for managing his care.

Skilled Nursing Facilities

Nursing homes are more commonly known as skilled nursing facilities (SNF's), but you may also hear the term rehabilitation center or acute care. It is not uncommon for someone to discharge to a skilled facility for recovery after a hospital stay. Most of the time these are short-term stays, but there are cases where longer or permanent stays are required for medically complex cases. Their staff usually consists of RN's, LPN's and CNA's who are available 24-hours.

Once someone no longer requires care from doctors and nurses in the hospital on a daily basis, he or she naturally wants to go home. For the course of treatment, though, extended care in a long term-care facility may be recommended by a hospital social worker or discharge planner. The social worker evaluates the needs of the patient, taking many factors under consideration such as: support that can be provided at home, home health service that requires an order from the doctor for intense physical therapy, occupational therapy, or in my mom's case, nursing support or placement in a skilled facility where the patient receives around-the-clock care. These facilities are not exclusive to seniors. Many other folks are in there. People who are recovering from catastrophic injuries that need rehabilitation will likely spend time in a skilled facility. The same exit process happens at the skilled facility as it does in the hospital. Once the patient has improved to the point where they are no longer benefiting from the daily supports, a discharge plan is put in place. It is common for the facility to request a discharge meeting so everyone is on the same page. If this is not scheduled, I highly recommend that you ask the discharge planner for a meeting at least three days prior to going home. In some cases, a social worker will even visit your parents' home before they are discharged to make sure you have all the supports in place for health and safety.

If your parent is going to a skilled nursing center after a hospital stay, be sure to confirm all costs you are responsible for covering. What will insurance cover, what does Medicare or Medicaid pay, and what you are responsible for paying?

Foster care

Foster homes are private homes with an average of four to 10 residents living in one house. They are staffed 24 hours a day and the services offered vary by state depending on rules and regulations. Foster care can be a less expensive and more home-like setting. Often, the rooms and common areas are shared. The shared environment creates more of a family environment and can be suitable for folks needing long-term assistance.

Your home

For some of us, having mom move in doesn't require a second thought, but there are a few things I think everyone should consider, such as your person's physical and mental condition. Usually, when parents are moving out of their own homes, it is because they are no longer able to live independently. You may feel like it's no problem—it's your duty even—to have your loved one live with you, especially after all he or she has done for you. But it's crucial to be realistic with how much care he or she will need, and how much you can give.

Consider your current schedule, your relationship with your parents, and your home itself. Do you have a room that will accommodate his or her needs? Will you need to install grab bars? Can you take on the additional expenses? Is your spouse in favor of the situation? Your kids?

I'm not trying to deter you from taking your parent in, but it's important to think through how this will impact your family before rushing into a situation.

CHAPTER FIVE

WHEN IT IS DEMENTIA

Besides the hundreds of clients I had with my in-home care company, I had a personal journey with dementia. My dad went from a perfectly healthy man-of-the-hour to a frustrated, violent, crazy person with dementia, living in a memory care facility, which in his mind was like a jail. My brother, Chris, since I was estranged from my dad, took on a lot of the tasks related to my dad's care, but I was in the sidelines making many other decisions.

I was often thrown by discoveries of how sick my dad was without us knowing it. People who have been leaders and drivers in their lives tend to hide and pull back when they start to get sick. For instance, if June runs the book club, and she thinks something is not right and she is not remembering, she will pass the club over to another person and hide. They don't want to get caught making a mistake. Now they lose skills faster, and it can be as simple as eating with a knife and a fork. I recall my dad's caregiver saying he wasn't hungry, but he would make him dinner anyway before he left. He peaked back through the window blinds and saw my dad did eat, but without utensils. He ate with his hands. My dad didn't want anyone to watch him eating. He loved cheeseburgers, but now he wanted to eat them day and night since there are no utensils required to scarf down a burger. I bought boxes of Angus Burgers at Costco and he would devour them in a few days. I know this was not the healthiest meal choice but I did not care as long as he was eating and it made him happy. Living with dementia is difficult enough; fighting over food choices was a battle I did not want to fight.

Your parent is the same, but he or she is different. The disease is now talking over. With The Devoted Daughter, I help sons and daughters deal with parents who can't verbalize how they feel when they are confused by the various stages of dementia. Your parents know something is wrong with them, but they can't put their finger on precisely what is happening to them emotionally at the time or why. They are going through brain failure, and it will kill you if something else doesn't; and there is no cure.

Parents who are living with dementia-related illnesses may exhibit behaviors ranging from anger, sadness, frustration, and many more. The brain is failing, so they are doing the best they can with what they have. They have lost executive functioning. You can often become frustrated thinking that your parent is acting irrational or emotionally erratic on purpose. Frustration is especially prevalent when your parents start asking the same question ten times in ten minutes or claim they have done self-care like showering when they haven't—they have lost their sense of smell and showers freak them out. They also get very argumentative about already paying bills or claiming rotten food is good. They are also wasting your time, and you have an agenda, so the parent and the kid are pushing against each other. You have a life and a time schedule, and they push against you.

At The Devoted Daughter, we provide a helpful guide to break tasks down into simple, slow steps with combative parents. It's possible you always had a combative relationship with your parent, so now it is crucial to not fall into the argumentative trap. Instead of muscling through, we help you feel supported and not alone in your preparation of tasks that can seem tedious on your own. We can help you to prepare to meet you parents in the middle. Let's take showering to show an example of breaking tasks and communication down into steps with your parents.

- You can give your parent the advice of the third party. "The doctor said the skin on your back is really dry, so we should shower and cream it."
- You can soak their feet to warm them up to the idea of bathing.
- You can wrap warm towels around their shoulders and put one in their lap, so they are not cold when they take their clothes off. Create an environment that is warm and inviting.
- You can buy a hand-held shower and a wand, so the water is not splashing everywhere, and you can control the water. A shower chair is great.

When I had my in-home care company, one of my clients lost his father suddenly. His mom was living with dementia and his sister was severely handicapped. There was always a tremendous amount of love in this family, but there was also the constant bantering between my client and his mother.

Jose's Story

"It took all hands on deck to figure out how to keep my mom and sister at home safely. I didn't want to tease and needle her, but I was unsure how to handle this new version of my mom who used to be able to handle the dynamic. She would start talking in Spanish. I knew she had dementia, but I struggled to accept it. She would do something that agitated me, and I would again feel like a 16-year-old boy fighting with my mom. I didn't know how to accept her limitations. She was always good at taking care of all my needs. I struggled to find activities for my mom that would make her feel proud and in charge. She was always a productive woman and worked very hard for every nickel. We had birds growing up and I thought it would be a good idea for her to watch over my birds when I was out of town. She always loved the birds, but when I brought them over for her to watch while I was out of town, she freaked out with the noise and seemed confused. One of her caregivers had to remove the birds from her house to keep them safe. I was at my wits end; she was not able to understand or process information in the same way. It was sad for me."

~~~~

As people age, they start unloading baggage they have been carrying around, or have they? Our parents have lived long lives. They have been through many ups and downs. Now they are in a health crisis and challenged in a way that creates more fright and fear. Amid their confusion about the changes in their health—mind and/or body—they are suddenly wrestling secrets that have been buried for years.

You are unsure of the validity of some of the truths they are dumping out. It is called confabulation, and it can be very challenging as a son and daughter because it is connected some times to your past also. Something from a TV show, something from the NY Times, and maybe a piece of something real is in there, and they will tell a story. They are owning it like it is their own life. How do you handle this new information? What you don't do is call them on the carpet and say it's not true or tell them that they are mixed. My dad would tell stories about stuff and I would hear rumors through the grapevine only to later find out if was not true.
~~~~

I understand that sometimes you even get disgusted at your parents and here is where you don't want to exchange words you will regret.

The Devoted Daughter has a lot of resources to help you cope with dementia and the feelings related to the challenges. Here is a ready list of solutions for the dementia mindset that will keep you out of frustration.

- Just agree with your parent. So what if they think the sky is red? Arguing is the worst. "No, John isn't coming today. He is coming tomorrow. I have told you that sixty times."
- You may find it difficult to agree to something that is not true, but she probably won't remember that tomorrow.
- Create breaks from your parent. I know for some people that is easier said or done, but find the advocate or that person from church who can give you a break. Don't feel guilty that you want to pass your parent off on someone else. If you don't fill up your own cup, you don't have much to give. Taking care of your parent will be less than a chore.

Some parents don't use their voice anymore, and they will stand and watch TV. You look in their eyes and they are empty. It is very sad. As a son or daughter, you have to give yourself the break to process your feelings of losing a parent. He or she is alive but you are losing him or her piece by piece.

People can also become mean to the person who is taking care of them, and that is hard to handle. A parent who has dementia is suddenly as mean as a snake.

By the time my dad was very sick, there was a lot of bad history between us. While my dad had many natural gifts—intelligence, athleticism, good looks, and a thriving dentistry practice—he lacked confidence, especially in social situations. He never got over not knowing his true identity. When my parents went to get their wedding license, my dad was unable to find his birth certificate. He discovered that his biological father was not the man he knew as his father. By that time, he found out his biological father had passed away. My mom said he was never the same after. The way he managed was with a professional persona and a private persona. His patients loved him, and he was generous with his time and concerned for the well-being of others, but often this was not the same man who came home every night to my mom. My older brother and I are three years apart, and my younger brother is fourteen years younger than I. My younger brother said to me that David and I were raised by a different dad. I had never thought of it that way, but he was right. By the time my younger brother was born, my parents were on the path to divorce.

I struggled with my relationship with my dad in my early twenties. He was involved in a new relationship and my parents loathed one another. It was not my fault they were divorced; why did I have to beg for his attention and time? My mom hosted a beautiful party before my wedding, and invited my dad. I remember the disappointment when he did not show up, and he did not call. After everyone left, I got in my car at 11:00 PM and drove to his house. He was shocked that I had the guts to confront him. He broke down in tears, apologizing for not going and somehow tried to blame my mom. I was angry and hurt, and I did not know what to do with those feelings, so I buried them deeper than the disappointment. At this point, I did not know if he would show up on my wedding day. My gram said to me, "Jackie O's dad did not show for her wedding." I was thinking, *I am not Jackie O and I need and want him to be there for me and everyone else.* He did show after all.

At The Devoted Daughter, we prompt you to consider the back story of your family. We help you break down the relationships of the past and acknowledge how that impacts the decisions you need to make now as your parents age.

My dad re-married and started a new family. We were all expected to respect his decisions and play a part in his new life. I thought this was crap! I was always polite and tried to have a semblance of a relationship, but it always felt obligatory. Nothing just flowed; naturally, there always had to be a reason to call or get together. I spoke to my mom several times a day for no reason. It was not that way with my dad.

My dad and I continued to have difficulty communicating. He called when he wanted something, and seemed to be angry that I spent so much time with my mom. I don't know what he expected; he left us, we did not leave him.

There are times when you have to set boundaries to protect yourself. I was at the point where I did not trust him with my emotions. What would be next? I did not think I would ever see him or speak to him again. Over the years, there were family events and a few dad sightings, but nothing substantial. My brothers were still speaking to my dad, and it was hard to be the black sheep of the family. I was no longer attending Christmas dinner, and I was not allowed to see my half-sister. Asking me to leave the family was his way of resolving the issue. God forbid we could talk about what had happened.

My dad wanted to continue to live on the coast. His living conditions were deplorable, but as long as he was safe, we would honor his wishes to stay there. Many community members who brought him food offered to help. He was reluctant to accept help and insisted he was fine. In the fall, he finally agreed to move back to Portland. My brother, Chris, was still on speaking terms with him and offered to rent him an apartment close to his home so he could look in on him. I decided to help my dad through

Chris. I had cared for my mom, and I knew how hard it was, and I did not want Chris to go through it on his own. Due to our estranged relationship, I never saw my dad during this time.

The decision to help in this way was something I could accept. Every family is unique, and only you can decide the best course of action for your family. Using the Circles of Care at The Devoted Daughter will help you identify and uncover what is best for your family.

Since I owned a home care company, I started to look for someone to help my dad. I knew he needed more support and that it would need to be the right person. If you have found yourself between a rock and a hard place, start asking people if they know anyone who can help. Don't give up; you might not find the right person out of the shoot. You may find that different people work better on different days or at different times of day.

We were not sure how long he had been living with dementia, but it was long enough to make a mess of his finances, communication with friends and family, and the ability to care for himself. Before long, it was clear he needed more help to be able to stay in the apartment. I got busy finding caregivers who could help with meals, transportation, medication, and Luther, the standard poodle. I didn't want the caregivers I hired to know it was my dad. I wanted them to remain professional and follow the rules as if they were working with any other clients. We also engaged Meals on Wheels, and although their mission is to provide homebound seniors with meals, they also offer human contact that so many seniors are missing. As it turned out, the couple who delivered my dad's meals had attended the same college as my dad and remembered him from his days on the basketball court. This was amazing because my dad had forgotten his education and his professional background, so they were able to relate to him on a topic he could still pull from his memory.

We soon learned that Luther was enjoying the meals on wheels, but we decided to keep the service. I knew the foods my dad enjoyed, so I started doing the shopping, cooking, and coordinating the supply chain. I dropped off care boxes with the food labeled and with clear instructions for cooking. The caregivers picked up the boxes at the apartment office and made sure my dad had what he needed. One afternoon, I was dropping off the box and I ran into the caregiver. The caregiver recognized me from the photographs in my dad's apartment. I explained a little bit about our history and asked him to keep me in the loop. From that day forward, Dwaine worked day and night helping my dad and our family until the day he died. I can't tell you what a godsend it was to have someone I trusted to help with the day to day. For me, it was my way of helping and honoring my dad without personally interacting with him.

My dad's ability to think was getting worse. He was wearing layers of clothing in 90-degree weather and turning on the heat instead of the air-conditioning. Health and safety were becoming more of a concern. He was also becoming combative and more confused. Late on a Thursday afternoon, my cell phone rang, and it was Dwaine. He was at my dad's house, and he was unable to communicate with him. Dwaine described him as weak, confused, and did not know what to do. I asked him to get him something to drink and see if that helped. He called me back about a half hour later and said he was getting worse. I told him to call 911, and I would call Chris and let him know that they were going to evaluate him and possibly take him over to the hospital.

The EMT's came and my dad became very combative. Dwaine suggested that they approach him differently, but the situation got worse instead of better. Eventually, the police were called and he was taken to the ER for evaluation. It was not an easy process and it could have been accomplished with less resistance had the emergency personnel been trained to handle people living with dementia. My dad remained in the hospital for several days and we knew there was no way he could continue to live independently; we would have to put him in memory care. During his time in the hospital, the staff could not get him to cooperate. Chris stayed with him during the night, but he was still pushing back. Dwaine was finally able to get him in the shower after promising him that he could leave soon. It was a full court press to get him to do anything. He kept talking about the dog and when was he going to be able to see the dog. Behind the scenes, we were all looking at each other saying, *what are we going to do with the dog?* I had the dog and had taken him immediately to the groomer and the vet for evaluation. Luther was undernourished and needed some TLC. I could not give the dog to a new owner. It was everything my dad looked forward to, so I agreed to keep the dog. I was not sure what was going to happen, but I was now the proud owner of Luther, the standard poodle. My dad knew I had the dog and that seemed to satisfy him for the time being. Pets can be a lifesaver, but they can also be a burden for people living with dementia. Pet care and the elderly is one of the topics we discuss over at The Devoted Daughter.

The next few days and weeks were crazy. We found a memory care unit that checked all the boxes. None of this is easy, and it certainly was not done without a lot of thought and consideration. I wish I had The Devoted Daughter available to me then! He was not capable of living independently, even with care, during all of his waking hours. My dad was discharged to the memory care after about a week in the hospital. We did not have any other options.

Now that he was safe and sound at his new home, we had the task of cleaning out a two-bedroom apartment that was filled from floor to ceiling. Over the next couple weeks, we sorted, tossed, donated, and looked through mounds of debris. I found a small suede pouch with beading on the outside. It looked like a souvenir from a gift shop. Tucked inside was a list of names and phone numbers along with my dad's Medicare card that had been missing for three years. There was also a note inside that said, "My name." Next to that entry was my dad's name and birthdate. I had to take a seat and let this sink in for a few minutes. This must have been written years earlier; he must have known something was wrong, and that he was unable to remember his name.

The memory care facility was helping to keep my dad safe, but it was a hell hole for people waiting for dementia to rob them of their memories and eventually take their lives. Dwaine helped my dad get out for day trips, cheeseburgers, and really anything my dad was up to for a change of scenery. He was not always willing to leave, but when he was, Dwaine would get him out as much as possible. Luther visited every week and was greeted by my dad enthusiastically at first, but he started to lose the ability to even connect with the dog.

My dad had lots of visitors from both family and friends. It was hard for people to accept him in this condition. I think some of those people were freaked out by the change. Maybe they were thinking, "Could this happen to me?" I don't know, but many of them came once and did not return. It is hard to see someone whose mental status has made such a dramatic shift. Friends and family should be prepared before seeing someone who is living with dementia, especially if they have not seen one another in a long time.

One afternoon, the facility was redoing the flooring. One of the aids took my dad outside. When he came back and noticed one of his basketball memorabilia books was missing, he blew a gasket. This resulted in punching someone and causing a violent scene. He was taken to the hospital, medicated and restrained. Our medical teams are not prepared to manage these complex dementia cases, but that is a whole other story. Patients who are confused, agitated, and appear off the rails are often sedated and sent to a geriatric psych ward, if a bed is even available. If a bed is not available, they are medicated so the hospital staff can deal with their behaviors. The emergency room is not the place for a person living with dementia, but often this is the only option.

It was a hot summer day in July, and this was the beginning of the end. My dad was fighting the medical teams with all of his might when he wasn't knocked on his ass with medication. At one point, he said to Dwaine, "This is not working. I am done with this shit." He pulled out the IV and was put in intensive care. Chris was there daily and counseled with the physicians on staff who agreed that he was able to make this decision. The next day, he was admitted to hospice and was transferred back to memory care for comfort measures. He was gone in a couple of days. I have heard people say you go out as you lived. He always wanted to be in control, and he was not going to have someone keep him alive just for the hell of it. As a family, we supported this decision, as none of us would want to live our lives waiting to die and be trapped in our minds.

Please remember that symptoms could appear that make it seem like your parent has dementia. Don't just assume. A friend called me the other day claiming her mom has dementia. I asked her if her hearing had been checked because I have seen her mom confused in social situations where there is a lot of background noise. She said no. I suggested that she should get her mom a good physical work up before assuming it was dementia. She was telling me that he mom speaks out of turn, repeats herself, and says things that are not relevant to the conversation. It may be that her mom is not getting input. My gram had hearing aids and would play along with the conversation like she knew what you were saying. When speaking on the phone became more difficult we set her phone up to utilize the speaker feature.

You can also try to re-phrase the way you are saying something to see if the other person picks up on the conversation. This would let you know that his or her hearing might be affected. She said her mom would be resistant to the hearing test, so I told her it might be a good idea to go have hearing tests together. It is always more fun with someone else along for the ride.

Dementia is increasing in numbers exponentially every year. According to the World Alzheimer's report, there are over **9.9 million new cases of dementia each year worldwide**, implying one new case every 3.2 seconds.

Watching your parents deteriorating is complex, layered, and not something you want to do alone. Check out The Devoted Daughter's site for updated preventative measures and information on dementia.

CHAPTER SIX

PAIN MANAGEMENT AND PROTECTION

In 2003, after Mom's hospitalization for emergency back surgery, she was placed in a skilled nursing facility. I realized very quickly that skilled nursing facilities were not always prepared to safely manage complex health care even though that was the sole reason she was there. Once you arrive, you are thrown into an unfamiliar setting with very sick people. I wanted to be polite; we needed these people to help my mom. I wanted to quickly ascertain who was in charge and who we would be speaking to about my mom's care.

Once we were assigned a room, I hustled to clean things up and get things organized. My mom could not see, so going into a new setting where you don't know where to find anything is overwhelming and scary. The first hurdle was that her medication orders were not correct. Once you leave the hospital, new orders are written and sent to the facility. The facility receives those orders and in turn orders the drugs from their contracted pharmacy. What happens if they don't have the medication? Red tape; that is what happens. If you do not double check, you may or may not get what was ordered. Don't assume that things are done correctly and don't be afraid to ask questions. At The Devoted Daughter, we give you a list of questions to ask when your parents are admitted to a skilled nursing facility from the hospital.

New medication orders are almost always written when someone leaves the hospital. Maybe you are accustomed to hearing the generic name of a drug versus the brand. Medications can be confusing so if you don't know *ask*, but how can you do that if you are sick as a dog? An advocate is vitally important when medical care is ordered. When you arrive at the facility, the first thing you want to do to is get your ducks in a row and find out who is in charge. You will need to know the names of the administrator, registered nurses who are responsible for caring for your parents, and other staff members you will interact with during your stay. I sat with the RN at the facility and went through all the orders one by one until we accounted for everything. When we realized the facility would not be able to get all my mom's medications, I went to my mom's house and got the medication she needed. They checked them in at the nurse's station, and the correct meds were administered from that day forward.

Getting my mom settled was not easy. She started having more pain in her leg, so she went back to the hospital for more tests where they found a blood clot. I did not know anything about this diagnosis. They did an ultrasound, and it looked to me like it would be a simple procedure. Oh my gosh, she was screaming in pain! I just broke down in tears; the technician assured me that it was painful and it was normal for her to be uncomfortable. My evaluation was that her pain level was far more than uncomfortable. Honestly, I found myself staring down a dark hole and wondering if I would ever see the light of day. The Devoted Daughter offers you insights and support when you are managing your parent's pain and you feel you cannot crawl out of a hole one more time. You deserve to have the support of others. You don't need to do caregiving alone. I know that is hard to believe when you're are in the midst of a family crisis, but you will be amazed how it feels when you connect with like minds. I was right where you might have been on the day we went back to the nursing home with more drugs and a new diagnosis, on top of everything else.

A few months later, my mom and I were back in the lobby of a skilled nursing facility waiting for her to be admitted once again. It was a rainy, dreary day, and it was the fifth time she had been through this in one year, so her spirits were quite low. I wanted to take her home then and there, but I knew it was more than I could handle. She was quite weak and needed 24-hour nursing care and physical therapy before she would be able to go home. Taking her home would mean that a qualified person would need to be awake around the clock and we would need to transport her to medical appointments. For those reasons, going home was not an option. Checking into this hell hole, a.k.a. the skilled medical facility once again was devastating for both of us. My mom and I had been down this road many times, so we were all too familiar with the process. All of a sudden, my mom burst into tears.

"Mom, are you ok?" I asked. "What is wrong?"

She looked at me, shaking, and said, "I am so confused, I can't think."

I knew she was scared and I was scared to death. There was no longer room for me to be a scared child. I had to be the adult in charge of my mom. I had to surmount my fear to understand what was happening for her at this moment. I needed the tools to guide me through this process. The Devoted Daughter has a checklist to break down the little shifts you can make when you are faced with a traumatic situation. What was bringing on this sudden confusion and sorrow now? I was thankful that she could verbalize her feelings, but it did not give me much comfort. I tried everything to reassure her that we would get her in a room and get her situated with all her things and figure out who the nurse on staff was. David and Sarah would be coming soon. Maybe they would be able to bring her granddaughter to visit tonight. She always lit up the room, and my mom worshiped her. Nothing seemed to help console her worries. I was racking my brain; what could I do to get her calmed down? I could not imagine how she was feeling. What could cause an overwhelming state of confusion? I did not have the answer, but I knew that if my mom had her family close, we would get through this awful day. Maybe that fearful obedience was kicking in now because I was not going to give up.

What I did not know at that time was that one of the aids had attempted to assault her in the middle of the night. She did not tell me until years later, and looking back, I have clarity into her fear. If only she had told me. By the time we did know, I had gone to the authorities and the management company of the facility. The person was no longer employed there, and they were unable to locate him. The fear in her eyes makes more sense looking back on the timeline. I had no way of knowing what had happened. I am still not sure why she did not tell me right away. We were there every day; maybe we could have stopped this person from hurting someone else. What kind of a dirtbag preys on the sick and the elderly?

What I did do was to make sure the presence of our family was known from that day forward. At The Devoted Daughter, we give you the tools and guidance to protect your parents. Yes, *you* are protecting *them* now. It is a big shift to accept. Anytime my mom was hospitalized, I would call the nurses' station at the beginning of each shift change and ask who was on duty. I also called again in the middle of the shift and at the end of the person's shift. I wanted them to know we were watching and paying attention. Often, my brother, David, would stay overnight with my mom. Although this may seem excessive, hospitals are no different than other service organizations, and the squeaky wheel gets the grease.

While I understand that hospitals are often understaffed and they are in a constant state of re-shuffling priorities based on patient needs, many times I felt like I was standing in front of the nurse's station with four nurses behind the desk talking about their personal lives. How could they be completely oblivious that someone was standing in front of the counter waiting for assistance? I am not bashing nurses, as we have had incredible care over the years. I am stating this because it happened over and over again. If it happens to you, I want you to be empowered to speak up. I am not talking about being a pest, but instead getting the help you need when you need it. There were many times when I thought to myself, *Screw it. I will just do it myself.* I was not going to let my mom suffer because someone was too busy socializing. Nursing is demanding, and many times a thankless job, and I can imagine there are times when they have to separate themselves emotionally to be able to continue to serve in that role. You never know what will be coming at you and many times it is life and death.

When my mom was in the hospital, I introduced myself and let the staff know who might be visiting. There is usually a whiteboard in every room. I would write down our names, relationship to my mom and contact information. I also had them make a sign and put it above my mom's bed, so everyone knew she was blind. Since her medical condition was complicated and she could not see, I always requested a room close to the nurse's station. It was important that she could call for help if needed. I always asked for the additional help my mom needed. It takes guts to stand up for yourself. A healthy dose of arrogance helps. A hospital is a place where people are staffed to help, and people are often screaming for help in tandem!

There were people who my mom did not want to see, mainly when she was critically ill. Since my mom was such a social person, her friends thought she would enjoy visitors during every hospital stay. When you are not feeling well and you look like hell, it is not the best time for a social call. I finally spoke to the charge nurse and told her my mom is not up to any visitors except family. We closed the door and put a sign on the door saying, "No visitors. Please inquire at the nurse's station." That caused the phone to ring off the hook, but thank goodness for silent mode.

When you have a parent who is sick, you need someone on your team who can advocate for you. Choosing the right person is important, and at The Devoted Daughter we provide you a checklist of questions to ask if you need to hire and advocate or nominate someone in your family. After all, this is a human being we are taking care of here! People will spend all kinds of money in the personal development of a human being, but then they hedge on hiring an advocate for their not-well parent.

There was one night that was the lowest moment in all the time my mom was sick. I had never felt so powerless. You believe you have to be so strong and fight, but an incident will just throw you. My mom had been taken to the hospital by ambulance for extreme back and leg pain. A lot of people don't consider how hard it is for someone to be transferred when sick. Think about it. You are laid out on a gurney with metal rails. You have people on both sides of you; outside the lights are flashing and sirens are blaring. I have not personally had this experience, but my mom told me that you could feel every bump in the road. For someone who is in that much pain, getting to the hospital was torture. Once we arrived, I was hoping she would be taken back to the emergency room immediately, but that was not the case. My mom was laid out on that gurney for what seemed like an eternity. She was pleading for help, and all I could do was be there and ask how much longer. I was sobbing quietly in despair. The staff seemed preoccupied and not concerned. I don't know what was happening that night, but from my perspective, it was unacceptable. When we were finally taken back, they wanted to give my mom morphine via injection. I knew she was sensitive to morphine and asked them to inject the drug slowly so it would not make her nauseous. After hours in the emergency room, they decided to admit her to the hospital. Once we got to her room, David and I were there and they were attempting to get her transferred from the gurney to the bed. The pain was off the charts and they gave her more morphine; sure enough, she started to vomit. All of a sudden, lights were going off and the staff was hustling around the room. My mom was sobbing in pain and David and I were asked to leave the room. My mom's blood pressure was dropping to unsafe levels; we could be losing her right before our eyes. I was in shock, and at that moment, I was grateful for the professionals who were stepping up, making decisions and transferring her to the intensive care unit. That is all we knew. Nothing more, nothing less. If you find yourself in a desperately frightening medical emergency, stay calm and do the best you can to advocate for your parents. I believe our constant presence and persistence saved my mom's life. It was not perfect, and it scared me to death, but we got through it.

I could not help but wonder if all this could have been avoided had she been seen hours earlier and they were able to control the pain. I was shaking, trying to be strong, but scared to death at the same time. There was also some comfort in knowing that there would be two nurses around the clock, keeping their eyes on her. Maybe we could get to the bottom of this once and for all. Deep down, I knew that was wishful thinking, but I wanted my mom to experience life without pain. They kept her in the intensive care unit for the next three days until her blood pressure returned to normal levels. Once she was back in her hospital room, we attempted to break down what had happened and why. To this day, I don't know what caused this chain of events.

As my mom's health became more complex and new ailments were discovered on a regular basis, communication between healthcare providers was essential. Her blood pressure was fluctuating and her kidneys were failing. Her doctors needed to understand the entire picture to treat her appropriately. My sister in law came to me one day in the hospital and said, "Your mom needs a primary care doctor." I brushed her off, thinking *she doesn't need one more person I have to update and go through to get care done.* At the time, primary care was not mandated for referrals and everything like it is today. Sarah suggested a clinic nearby that specialized in concierge service. There is an annual fee, but they offer a higher level of service to their patients. I agreed to check it out, and we made an appointment for the following week. I was so relieved to hear that not only would my mom have more resources at her disposal, but I now had someone who I could call and ask questions to, update, and coordinate care. Having more personal care was definitely a bonus and saved my mom from the unnecessary hospital and skilled nursing stays.

When someone is in and out the hospital with many different specialists evaluating their health, you need the whole picture. That is not to say you are treating every aliment at once, but it is necessary for rotating physicians to understand the baseline of their patients. I was not always sure what information was most important, so my brothers and I researched and asked everyone we knew for information that might help my mom's medical condition. One of the benefits of having the concierge doctor was to collaborate and bounce ideas off a team of medical professionals. The team was also able to access test results and medical updates in real time, so we did not have to endure waiting anxiously for hours. At The Devoted Daughter, we offer suggestions to help you build the medical support resources you need for your family. They can be organized in one of your circles of care.

Once you have exhausted all the resources of traditional medicine, then what? We were holding onto hope and praying my mom would find some relief from the pain. Her medical situation was becoming more complex each day. Everyone in the family was grasping at straws to find a solution that could help with the pain. We spent endless hours researching, making calls, and calling in any favors from anyone who would listen. I was taking my mom to what seemed like a new doctor every week. We were finally able to get an appointment with a well-known physician at a pain clinic; he was known for forward thinking and medical trials. At this point, my mom was unable to walk due to the pain. She was able to bear some weight and transfer from standing to a wheelchair. She had already gone through so much and becoming unable to walk was another blow that was very discouraging. We arrived at the hospital for the appointment, and I assisted my mom out of the car and into the transport wheelchair. Transport chairs are a great alternative to a bulky, heavy wheelchair. The chair folds up and fits into the trunk of a car and is easily assembled. Go to The Devoted Daughter for suggestions on how to access durable medical equipment and other medical supplies.

I got my mom situated in the wheelchair and we were just getting on the elevator when she announced, "I am in trouble, here comes diarrhea." Oh my gosh, we have been waiting months for this appointment; now what?

"It's going to be fine, mom," I said. "We will figure out how to get you cleaned up, but we were not going to miss this appointment come hell or high water." Luckily, in that instance, I had learned through trial and error that helping someone who is chronically ill who can't walk or see and has immense pain takes time. When we needed to be somewhere at a specific time, I planned for an extra two hours to get there and back. As you work through your own circles of care, you will see how important planning is to get the necessary care and to reduce stress.

Diabetes had given my mom another blow. Over time, high glucose levels in the blood can cause the arteries to harden and restrict blood flow to the heart. By-pass surgery was not for the faint of heart, no pun intended, and for her, it was risky because of her pre-existing health problems; yet, she had to have the surgery to survive. I was confident in the surgeon, as he came highly recommended. We all agreed that this was the best option for my mom, but I could not help but think, should we be getting a second opinion? We had already waited for months to get to see this doctor and go through all of the preliminary steps. My mom was anxious to have the surgery and be done. The morning of the surgery, we were all at the hospital. It was early, around 6:00 AM, and they put us in a pre-op room. I knew this was a big surgery, but it did not hit me until the priest from the hospital visited us. That sent me over the edge. I had never been through this, so I did not know what to expect. This was a Catholic hospital and a priest was part of the process, but who knew? In my typical mindset, I was thinking, don't borrow trouble. We are ok right now. Let's see how this plays out and we will take it from there. My mom went to ICU just after surgery and stayed there for a couple days. The recovery was especially brutal due to my mom's fragile state. She remained in the hospital for at least a week and then went to a skilled nursing facility until she was well enough to return home. I had many instances with my mom where she was in surgeries and procedures. I was powerless over how she felt or recovered. I sometimes could not even persuade her to do what I knew was better for her overall health, and she further suffered.

I witnessed my mom experiencing so many instances of pain, I wanted to find a solution to the pain. The pain was the bull's eye on the wall, and we needed to attack it from every angle. We attempted non-tradition solutions such as acupuncture and chiropractic care. For those of you who are thinking that non-traditional approaches are for the birds, you most likely have not been in a desperate situation. I would have tried anything to help my mom, but that is not to say that this self-care shouldn't have started long before our backs were against the wall. If she had started moving her joints and spine before the pain was debilitating, maybe she would have had better long-term results.

The pain clinic offered services from 'a team of professionals. I found the holistic approach to treating the entire person to be refreshing. To qualify, you had to meet with a psychiatrist. My mom would have done anything to get some relief from the pain. Imagine being in so much pain that you can't get out of bed, take a shower, or pick up around the house. Over time, you are beaten down and many people become clinically depressed.

The pain clinic wanted to make sure they were treating the entire problem. The evaluation was extensive, especially when evaluating all her medications and the potential for drug interactions. They were able to recommend some outside resources for exercise and pain relief. My mom started working with a physical therapist in the pool. At last, there was a therapy recommendation for something she enjoyed and could look forward to attending. Getting to and from the pool was not easy due to her eyesight and instability in her gate. We put together a swimming bag with all the necessary items. I wanted this to be fun for her. Next, we established a routine for her to put her suit on at home and pull on sweats over the top, so she could get in and out of the pool with the least amount of effort. Within three weeks, she started to see some improvement. Swimming allows you to move and still be supported by the water, and it puts the least amount of stress and strain on the body. Much of the pain my mom was experiencing was nerve pain, so they decided to enroll her in a clinical trial for an anti-depressant drug that had been found to work on nerve pain. Drugs can be developed for a specific purpose, but they can also be effective for treating unrelated medical conditions. Once she was accepted into the trial, it would take six months before the FDA would approve the drug for distribution. The combination of new drug therapy, chiropractic care, and movement was helping her feel better. The good news was she was finally able to throw in the towel on the wheelchair! It felt like we were making progress and now there was hope and light at the end of what seemed like a long, dark tunnel.

CHAPTER SEVEN

NEVER READY TO DIE

My mom wasn't ready to die. Whoever is? How do you prepare for something like a parent's death when all you have been doing is working to keep them alive?

Just when I thought we were making some headway with my mom's pain management and her health, she started complaining of stomach pain that was radiating into her back. She was already on dialysis, but then we received the dreaded diagnosis of pancreatic cancer. She went in for what we thought would be a routine scan to try and figure out the source of the stomach pain. It was early January, and the results of the scan would be available in a week or so. We had no idea what to expect, but at this point, she had endured so much that who the heck knew?

January 16th, my brother's birthday. The snow was coming down and everyone in Portland was trying to get home as quickly as possible to avoid traffic mayhem. The phone rang around 4:00 PM and my mom was hysterical. I could hardly understand what she was saying. The surgeon had called my mom on the phone and informed her that she had pancreatic cancer. He did not offer an I am sorry or any compassion when he delivered the news of this terminal diagnosis. What the hell?! Who in their right mind would call a medically fragile patient during a snowstorm and drop this bomb? I was incredulous at this behavior. How would he feel if someone did this to his mom, sister, or daughter? I guess I will never know. I could have called him and unleashed my anger, but I had learned very well by now to pick my battles. My mom was who needed me at this moment, and once I got over the shock, I focused on getting to her house regardless of the weather. I lived across town at the time, but David said he was going to get over there and pick up my mom for dinner and spend some time with her to make sure she was okay for the night. David and Sarah found my mom weeping in despair. What would happen next?

First thing in the morning, I contacted my mom's primary care physician at the concierge medical clinic. We were able to get in touch with them right away, which continued to be one of the benefits of this service. He looked up the test results and confirmed the dreadful news. He was very familiar with all my mom's health challenges, and that positioned him to be an excellent advocate. We identified some of the most highly respected oncologists in our area. Time was critical, so we knew the ball needed to get rolling. Pancreatic cancer is difficult to treat with surgery, and based on my mom's health, operating was most likely not an option. I wanted to learn as much as possible about next steps and how this would impact her current treatments. She was already in renal failure and dependent on dialysis three days a week.

None of us wanted her to opt for chemotherapy. We met with the oncologist and he outlined the options. The meeting was tense and scary. We sat there, listening on the edge of our chairs, as he presented us with options, and none of them sounded good. The chance of making it out alive was slim. We all asked questions, but this was my mom's decision. The doctor was very kind and empathetic, a complete juxtaposition from the surgeon we met with earlier in the month. He told my mom about a woman he had been treating for five years. She was having success with a new chemotherapy drug. He gave my mom her phone number and told her that it might be helpful to talk with someone who was going through treatment.

Leaving the meeting, I felt very discouraged. When your body is already broken and you are going to put poison in it on top of everything else, the odds of winning the fight are slim to none. If it were my choice as a super sick person, I would have opted to let nature take its course and live a better quality of life in the time I had left. My mom, though, did not want to leave us. She was ready to fight, and it was her choice.

When your parent makes an ultimate decision about his or her body, you should cast no judgment.

Here is where he or she is an adult, and so are you. As a devoted daughter, I was accustomed to taking the lead. The mindset of doing the right thing and protecting my mom was foremost in my mind, but her courage reminded me that she was the leader of the pack. You can quickly fall into the role of caregiver and forego your role as a daughter or son. If I had one regret through this process, it was assuming the role of caregiver and too often forgetting that I was her daughter. I was so amazed at her bravery. *How does she do it?* Around every corner, something was trying to knock her down, and she just kept fighting back.

The next morning, my mom placed a call to Jerry, the chemo patient, to learn more about her experience with the chemo treatments. Jerry told my mom that it was not a picnic, but she was alive and overall doing well. Since surgery was not an option, my mom felt like her only chance at beating this was to have the chemotherapy treatment. The side effects of the drug could be fatal. It was a delicate balance to administer the chemotherapy and continue dialysis treatments. Since she was in renal failure, the chemotherapy dosage would need to be monitored and adjusted, based on kidney function. That afternoon, my mom announced she was ready to proceed with the chemo and wanted to make her first appointment. She loved life and wanted to spend time with her family and her friends. It was hard to see someone so full of life being faced with the better-bad choice to survive.

I was so focused on the task at hand that I failed to consider the benefits of including others in her treatment plan. Some of my mom's friends could have taken her to chemo. Then after they spent time with her, they could have the privilege of getting on the hotline to update the girls. The treatment lasted three hours and my mom loved listening to stories about other people's children and grandchildren. Companionship and support would have meant the world to her. You have the opportunity to make this adjustment if you have a loved one going through chemo.

The first morning of her chemo treatment, we arrived early for all the ins and outs, dos and don'ts from the nursing staff. They braced us for side effects, but they could not be sure what would happen; everyone reacts a little different. My mom already had a port in her neck for dialysis, so they would use that port to administer the chemotherapy as well. We started off with what would be a regular drill from this day forward: arrive, weigh in, take blood pressure, see the nurse practitioner, and go back to the infusion room for treatment. I had quit my other job, so I had more time, but I was also starting a private endeavor for in-home care.

On the way home, my mom was weak and starting to show signs of the drug taking over. I was nervous as a cat, and I wanted to get her home and tucked into bed. I thought if I could get her comfortable it would be okay. Boy, was I wrong! By the time we walked in the door, she was vomiting uncontrollably. What the hell was I thinking?! While no one could have explained how bad this could be, I should have hired professional help to get us through the transition. If it had been easy and drama free (which it wasn't), then at least I would have covered my bases. My mom's body was so fragile that trying alone to help her and moving her around to change her clothing and clean her up could have put her in harm's way. I just wanted to get her back to whatever kind of normal we could find. I encourage you to consider having a support system in place. If you don't need it, no harm no foul, but if you need help and you don't have it, you don't want to have to deal with the crazy mess I encountered. I have never smelled such an awful smell. The drug was oozing from her pores, and the stench was permeating the entire apartment. I could not clean up fast enough, and it kept coming. I had to get her clothes off, and I knew she was in pain, so I grabbed a pair of scissors and cut them off. The washer and dryer were in the front of the apartment next to the door so everything that I could wash was going in the laundry and everything that was too soiled was going outside in a garbage bag. I finally got her into bed and cleaned up. She was in so much agony. Since there was no guarantee of the outcome of this treatment, I could not help but wonder if this was worth it, but I was committed to supporting my mom through this time. She was determined, and she chose to be brave and to do everything she could to stay alive. Her family would be there by her side through thick and thin no matter how hard it was to watch her go through the treatment.

The following week we were given an infusion schedule. Some weeks would be more terrible than others, but at least we had an idea of what the next couple months would entail. Blood tests for cancer markers would be done on a scheduled basis to identify whether the treatment was effective. These tests detect chemicals in the blood made by tumors. That allows the oncologist to modify or change the dosage as needed. The side effects of the drug continued to be problematic. Nausea and oral thrush were the worst. Oral thrush is white and red open sores in the mouth and throat. The ulcers were treated with an oral rinse, but that made it hard to swallow, and food did not sound appetizing. I started working with a nutritionist in the oncology department to be sure this was not impacting her overall health. They suggested several protein powders, frozen fruit, and yogurt combinations. My mom loved fruit and yogurt, so that sounded good to her, but getting it down was another story. Some days it would take over an hour to have just a few sips. We made a pact that she would try to eat and drink small amounts throughout the day. I had to make a conscious effort to follow the plan of care and not to run down the google rabbit hole. The nutritionists were experts in their field and at some point, I needed to stop second guessing everyone.

Nutrition is an essential part of chemotherapy treatment. You are not only dealing with cancer, but the side effects of treatment can be very uncomfortable. My friend and client Laura tells about her own breast cancer battle on the heels of losing her husband to cancer.

Laura's Story

"I hired in-home care to help with my mother. My husband's cancer was finally in remission and we wanted to spend some time traveling. In-home care was a blessing, and I was so excited to spend some quality time with Jim now that he was feeling better.

"A few months went by, and life was rolling along swimmingly until Jim's cancer returned with a vengeance. We lost him in a matter of weeks! During the last week of his life, I was diagnosed with stage four cancer. I called Kelli early one morning and said, "I need help." I will never forget the conversation, but I knew I could not do this alone and I did not want my children to have to go through the painstaking process of cancer treatment on the heels losing their dad.

"The treatment was rough. I had no appetite, and I felt like crap! Kelli suggested that we come up with some nutritional options to keep me hydrated and get something in my body so I could continue to endure the horrific treatment. The RN on her staff put together a few options. You never know what is going to sound good so it is wise to have a couple choices. Having solid food, hydration, and nutrition was a godsend.

"During the next few months, we stuck to the infusion schedule, despite the fact that we were not feeling too hopeful. The treatments did not seem to be making a difference. We had sparks of hope, and then the letdown followed. My children were there by my side every step of the way. I could not imagine their despair after just losing Jim and now me. I was not as concerned about my daughter, as we shared a spiritual connection, but my son was another story. He had taken over the family business and was quiet and stoic. I pray every day that he can find peace and happiness in his life."

~~~~

As we started to get into more of a routine, I would get my mom set up in her chair, and she would usually rest during the time of the infusion. That gave me an hour or so to run errands or get some work done. One afternoon, I returned to find my mom sitting next to an older gentleman. She was using a walker that was next to her chair. I greeted her and asked if she was ready to go? I would grab my mom around her waist in a bear hug position and say, "One, two, three…up we go." I then took her hands and placed them on the walker to make sure she was steady. As we were doing this maneuver, the man in the chair next to us looked up at me and said, "I wish I had someone to help me like you are helping your mom. She is very lucky."
~~~~

"I don't know about the lucky part," I said. "But we love her very much and would not have it any other way."

That got me thinking about all the people who did not have anyone. What do they do? Are they left to fend for themselves after their chemo treatments? For those folks who are going it alone, there are research support groups, volunteers through local senior centers, private caregiver companies, county and state senior services, and veterans' benefits. I could not imagine having to go this alone after what my mom went through. I could have hired someone, but I was not going to leave my mom with a stranger during this time. I was able to make the time, and this is where I wanted to spend my time. I know that is not always possible for everyone. The care and treatment were involved, but more importantly, it was personal. Up until now, I did not hire someone to come into the home and help my mom. We made due with friends and family, but it was starting to wear us down.

One day I woke up and thought, *I am going to be in that infusion chair next to my mom if I don't start taking time for myself.* I quit my job, and I was taking care of my mom full-time, not realizing the emotional toll it was taking on my life; I still did not see that hiring someone or asking for my help could have made a big difference. I did hire a personal trainer to help me stay committed to my fitness routine.

For once, I was accountable to someone who was helping me take of me. It is easier said than done, as the most urgent matters always rise to the top of the priority list. These are the times when you have to time-block non-negotiable time slots to do something for you. Even if that is going outside alone and breathing. As the saying goes, "You can't pour from an empty cup."

How do you help your family and continue to expand your resources when you need help with your sick parent? The time may come when you have to throw in the towel, and you can't do it all yourself. Managing different solutions for pain control and medicine is one area to tackle, but daily assistance can grow overwhelming and beyond your capacity.

Driving to appointments was becoming too much of a daily requirement for just David and me to handle. One day, I had dropped my mom off at a doctor's office, and I was going to park my car and go back to meet her. I noticed a sedan driving through the drop-off line, and it said, "Nancy's medical transport." I pulled over and jotted down the number. I thought finding someone to transport my mom to medical appointments would help take some of the pressure off, but I could not even get the company to return my calls. So much for that idea. I felt discouraged after finally making the decision that I needed help, and I was willing to make the call and pay for the service. Often, it would feel like there was a ray of sunshine and then it was dark. There had to be a better solution.

What I know now is that you may want to consider a service that offers more than transportation, like an in-home care company. My mom couldn't see and was medically too fragile to navigate transportation without some personal assistance.

My mom's wishes were to stay at home, and I wanted to honor that request. We called a few in-home and home-health companies and scheduled appointments. In-home care companies are typically non-medical and provide things like transportation, light housekeeping, and meal preparation, although the services offered vary by state. Home-health offers supervised skilled care in the home. Their service includes physical therapy, occupational therapy, wound care, etc. There is 24-hour nursing support and physicians on staff. They also write medical orders. Home health is a service that is prescribed by a doctor for those people who are housebound and cannot get to an outpatient setting for treatment. It is currently covered under Medicare with a prescription, and home healthcare will continue working with their patients until the patient is no longer benefiting or improving from the services they offer. Many people think that if they are discharged from home health that the benefit has ended. That is not true. Home health service can be reinstated if the patient qualifies for the assistance. My mom had experienced some help with the home health company and since they had the same team members on board for years, she always received Pam after hospital discharge. Pam came into my mom's life during a hard time and offered more than just physical therapy. My mom and Pam became friends. They shared stories about their kids, laughed together, and cried together. Sometimes unexpected friendships form during the worst of times. Friendships can be formed with your parent and his or her caretaker that takes the weight off you being the one to orchestrate all the joy. I encouraged my mom to accept help from others by saying, "You need someone else to bring something to the party."

Now, I needed to consider in-home care because I was planning on going out of town for a couple weeks. I knew I needed to find someone who could help her during that time. I thought about the in-home care agencies we interviewed, but my mom did not feel a connection with any of them, and after all, she was the one who would be spending her days with these people. At the last minute, one of my friends recommended a young nursing student named Aura. I asked Aura to meet with my mom and me. Aura was full of life and passionate about nursing. She was in her second year of nursing school at the time. My mom loved her, and it was a match made in heaven. We made the decision to hire privately, but keep in mind that you are taking on the responsibility of an employer. The rules and regulations vary by state. For the next few days, we went over the routine, I showed her where things were and put together my mom's medical documentation. During the time I was gone, I must have called a million times a day. Talk about an overprotective mother hen. I did not enjoy my vacation like I needed to.

Every time I called, they were either at Target, ordering coffee, or getting my mom's hair done and most importantly having a blast. Finally, a lightbulb went off in my head. Someone else can help, and my mom does not feel neglected in any way. In fact, my mom enjoyed Aura so much that she stayed on to help my mom for the entire summer. What a gift! Aura returned until she graduated, and she and my mom remained lifelong pals. Another example of a stranger who showed up in the right place at the right time.

For every family, knowing when it's time to get help varies. In my professional experience, I have helped hundreds of people through this process, and each one always has a unique twist. I recently met with a family who told me they were looking for a few hours of help a few days a week. His daughter said, "Dad is sharp as a tack, but he needs some more help around the house." Upon my arrival, I learned that he had congestive heart failure, cancer, high blood pressure, neuropathy, gout, he was a fall risk, and wears Depends for incontinence problems. I was not seeing the same man that was described to me on the phone. It was clear to me that his family worships him, and they want was is best, but some things struck me as a little bizarre. He is wearing depends because he is pooping his pants, yet he is no longer showering. His son tells me that his dad does not feel the need to shower. Sitting in your feces is a health and safety risk, but I had to pick my battles. I can't waltz in the door when I am meeting people for the first time and start demanding they change.

The same is true when dealing with your parents. If you try to change everything at once, you are most likely going to get pushback. Try starting with the items that are most critical and then tackle those piece by piece. Slow and steady wins the race; it does not have to be done in one day. Most of us don't have a lot of extra time, but trust me, if you do too much at once you may end up starting back at square one; and that takes more time than just slowing down in the first place. Keep in mind that this can be a time of life when people experience a lot of loss. Doing things their way in their home is still something they can control. It may not be the best way, but it is not your home or your life. I have found that by taking the approach of helping or doing things together has a much better outcome. Asking questions and learning why someone wants to do things a certain way can shed some light on how they are thinking. Once you gain insight into their thought process, you may also figure out a better way to work together.

Before you even get to this place, there are processes and resources to help you identify concerns about your parents early on. There is a lot of information out there, and people are quickly overwhelmed. The first thing I do is google something and then work backward. That is not always the best approach, especially when it comes to healthcare. There are many times when a person seeks medical care for one thing, but in the end, the diagnosis comes back with more than one ailment. Weeding through clinical websites can be like reading a foreign language. Some of the information may apply to your mom, but what about the missing pieces? How can you problem-solve and plan for what you have in front of you now and what's coming down the road? At The Devoted Daughter, I provide practical advice for the earlier steps, acknowledging your parents are needing more help and you have more urgent questions. The topic of caring for your parents is not something we think about every day when they are healthy and enjoying retirement. We can talk out how many weeks of help you need before you get to overwhelm mode.

CHAPTER EIGHT

IN-HOME CARE: BEYOND FAMILY

Ninety percent of seniors say they want to stay at home. My mom did. In fact, I built her a whole new house so she could be comfortable! Still, she needed people to help her. I found the in-home care company online at a time when my mom needed all my care; I quickly uncovered there was a gap in the marketplace for caregivers needed to help seniors remain independent at home. I wasn't working, and I saw the need, so I invested the money and time. I have no regrets about my choice because it launched a career running my in-home care franchise that spanned eleven years, and helped over one thousand families. It was a vast up-level of my knowledge base from just caring for my mom. My heart was all in. I went from caring for a family member to running a company of over one hundred employees. Without this experience, I wouldn't have been exposed to how many sons and daughters lost their coveted relationships with their parents in the overwhelm of their sickness, or the changes in their parents. I also know firsthand, at The Devoted Daughter, all the specifics on what to look for when choosing an in-home care company for your loved one.

There are two essential elements of an excellent in-home care provider. The first is the people working with your family. There are so many skills that can be taught, but you can't show someone how to be a good human. I would often tell families there are skills we can coach someone on and there are obstacles that are deal breakers.

Secondly, can the service provider meet your needs? Do they have employees who will show up and what are the contingency plans if someone is sick or their car breaks down?

I knew that I wanted to help others, but I was not interested in lots of paperwork, forms, and legal mumbo-jumbo. The franchise was flexible, and I was willing to grow and learn from others within the system. I got a lot of help with administrative support through the franchise system. It was an exciting time when I needed a new endeavor to get out of bed in the morning. I loved the concept, especially since in-home care was not a well-known industry.

Selecting an in-home care company

1. Make sure the owners are involved in the business and have experience. I had little or no experience running an in-home care agency, but I had extensive medical knowledge. After what I went through with my mom, no situation baffled me. In my agency, we dealt with many medically complex cases. Choose an agency for your parents that has a high level of information and medical experiences under its belt.
2. Some agencies are going to fail, and you don't want to align yourself or your family with a company that will fold. Many people I trained with were gone from the business in less than five years. You don't want to start a relationship with an agency and have them go out of business because then you have to start all over again. Don't be afraid to ask questions: Who works in their office? Who handles the scheduling? What happens after hours?

You should also be mindful of the type of work an agency performs. Every state has different laws when it comes to licensing. In some states, you don't even need a license to offer in-home care services. There are also states that offer you registries where caregivers can be hired privately from the list. Buyer beware; once you cross that line, you are now an employer. Are you prepared to follow all the rules and regulations? Do you have insurance in case of an accident or a worker's compensation issue? It is becoming more common for people to hire someone privately and offer room and board as a part of the compensation package. Once someone is living in the home, if they are not willing to leave voluntarily, you would have to evict them formally. Did you know that could take months or even years?

When I first started the business, people were lining up to be caregivers. Today, many agencies have waiting lists for care. Finding, hiring, training, vetting and retaining qualified candidates is more and more difficult. Start thinking about these scenarios now. You may be saying to yourself, "Why should I think about this now?" Well, it is never too early to prepare yourself and your family for what might happen in the future. Caregivers are in demand as our population ages. Learning more about who is willing to do what and knowing how your parents feel about their futures cannot happen soon enough. Investigate your parent's insurance. Does he or she have a long-term care policy? It is not getting any more accessible, and with a shrinking workforce, costs are going to increase significantly. The reason prices will increase is: There are so many rules and laws to follow in the senior care business. Most of those are designed to protect the seniors, but many of them are not. Many states are implementing higher minimum wage requirements. I was operating in an employee rights state, and that has its own set of challenges. Increased regulation comes at a higher cost to the end user. I can't tell you how many people have asked me "How much is the caregiver paid?" I would love to pay the caregivers more, but I have to pay the taxes, my office staff, and implement health and safety, all while keeping the service affordable. The margins are very narrow, and I will tell you that most people in this business are in it because they care about others and want to give back, not to get rich.

Many people think they have considered all their options when it comes to caring for their aging parents. The reality is that none of us has a crystal ball. Your family's circumstances can change on a dime. Planning for your parent's future is not an option; it is a necessity!

I have worked with many families who thought they had planned for their parents' future; after all, they talked with mom and dad about it last year. Mom and dad both agreed to take a look at moving when the time was right. Don't be surprised when they start making excuses and saying they will decide within the next five years. You thought they would consider a move in the next year and they are thinking five. You are not on the same page, now what? If you have not hired help yet, or have someone local to check in on your parent, here is a cautionary tale:

Debra's Story

"The physician of my mom, Betty, recently evaluated her and determined that she could no longer live at home by herself. My husband and I lived out of state but our son lived upstairs, so we thought he could be helpful. Turns out he was gone most of the time, so we needed more help. Yes, the house was unkempt and the yard was overgrown and brown, but it was hard to maintain her home and ours. We had no idea there was trash spilling out of the trash can in the carport, the front door was covered with cobwebs, and newspapers were filling the doorstep. Kelli reported this to us after a visit with our son. My mom lived in the basement, which had been converted into an apartment so she would not have to navigate the stairs. My husband and I had done the remodel for her during one of our visits. Kelli reported to me that the place was filthy! My mom had lost her sight several years back so she must not have seen the cat hair and dirt in the carpet. She never told us or complained, and our son never mentioned that the kitchen floor had a layer of mud and grease. There was an ironing board covered with medications in the kitchen. My mom had told us that she could see them and take them independently. Apparently, down the hallway that led to a washer/dryer, bathroom, and bedroom was stains of feces on the walls. The bathroom was covered in feces. There were soiled depends and filth everywhere. The bedroom was another horrible sight. The mattress was sitting on the floor and clothing was piled everywhere. In between the clothing was a nest of dirty Kleenex. It was heartbreaking to hear about this, and we got defensive at first because we would never reduce Betty to living in squalor.

"I insisted to Kelli that my mother had always been sloppy. Kelli, despite my resistance, cleaned the whole place and got to know my mom on her terms. As time went on, she started to gain strength and Kelli reported back to me that she was eventually able to walk to the mailbox and back. She had not been able to stand independently for years, so it was a significant accomplishment and something to celebrate. I am so grateful we allowed Kelli and her staff to take care of my mom because from out of town we had no idea what was happening."

The family agreed to 24-hour care seven days a week. At the time, we were able to have caregivers staying with Betty for two and three days at a time. The laws have changed. This service is more difficult to staff and, in many cases, not available. As I mentioned earlier, hiring an in-home care agency familiar with the current regulations is vital. Someone who can advocate alongside this hire is also crucial, especially if you have an aging parent located out of state, or your access to them is limited; in fact, even along with the caregiver, I would suggest having a couple people you trust put eyeballs on the situation. In this case, the grandson was neglecting his grandmother, and the family was unaware of the deplorable conditions. If there had been another family member or friend stopping by, he or she would have had more insight. There were also health and safety concerns with her medication. If possible, when directing care from afar, you should make an effort to visit. Knowing first-hand what is happening allows you a better foundation for your decisions. I can imagine hearing that brings up a whole slew of resistance and excuses, like your job, time management, and immediate family concerns, but the longer you don't take care of the circumstances of an aging parent, the worse the situation can get. Just because someone lived in a messy house all his or her life does not mean that he or she should be living in filthy, unsafe conditions.

~~~~

The cost of hiring private care is shocking. Many families never discuss caring for their parents until they are hit squarely between the eyes with a medical emergency or diagnosis. They are shocked to find out that Medicare will not cover all the costs for in-home care or that hospice does not stay with your parents 24/7 during the dying process. Start reviewing these costs today! You need to plan for your parent's future, and you cannot do that if you are living under a rock. Stats from the U.S. Bureau of Labor Statistics show a 38% jump in the number of jobs for home health aides from 2014 to 2024. According to the BLS there will be 1.2 million home health aides.

I am here to inform you what you are up against, and also to help you seek resources.
~~~~

You could be in a position of not being able to afford it as much as you need to. At The Devoted Daughter, we use the Circles of Care model to help you still have your life, but put into compartments everything you are going to be responsible for. We also help you to organize your parents' affairs so that when you do need to facilitate doctor's appointments, hospital visits, or administer medications yourself, order prevails. I lived a very chaotic existence while taking care of my mom, but then I learned all the right ways to care for the elderly through my in-home care company. I don't want you to go through what I did as a daughter. I want you to be able to retain the dignity of your birth-given role.

CHAPTER NINE

ORGANIZATION IS KEY

I spent years worrying every night about the sound of the phone ringing and what could happen to my mom. I was powerless over her destiny, waiting for the other shoe to drop. You don't need to live your life this way as a son or daughter who has caregiver responsibilities. There are strategies and tasks to prepare yourself for that unexpected call in the middle of the night. For starters, organizing paperwork and gathering information is phase one to having a less frantic experience with the emergency room. Do you have a list of current medications, emergency contacts, known allergies, and any details that could be helpful to a medical professional?

Medical paperwork and insurance information is a pain for anyone, but it's especially tricky when it's your parent's paperwork, and he or she hasn't made efforts to keep it in order. Organizing paperwork in a regular doctor's visit is far easier than digging through a stack of foreign medical documents in an emergency. I have heard horror stories from physicians in the ER saying people came in and had no idea what meds they were taking; they have no list. When it comes to surgery, you have to open them up and hope for the best.

Before you burst into your parent's homes to start getting them organized, understand they can be resistant. My gram had a whole system for her meds that frankly made no sense to anyone but her. She had everything in a shoe box. Inside the box were medication bottles with handwritten labels attached to the jars with rubber bands. She had little notes scribbled on pieces of paper with lines through medication that had been changed or discontinued. She was not interested in me coming in and creating a new system for her medication orders. You have to pick your battles. The idea of organizing paperwork can seem like a much bigger deal to your parents than to you, so before doing anything, talk with him or her about why you want to get the papers organized, and the importance of documentation accuracy.

If your parents have been hoarding, and trying to help them to get organized always ends in fights, this is a sign a more serious underlying problem could be developing. With any change, take it slow, with one step at a time. Imagine yourself in their shoes. Here is where you can be the compassionate son or daughter, and not just the hired caregiver. You have time for compassion, especially if other people are helping you with your parents' care. At times, it can feel like you are out of options, but The Devoted Daughter will offer you a myriad of ideas to work your way through the daily conundrums you face when helping your parents. We consider what is happening to you right now, and we are solution driven!

First, let's tackle the emergency folder so you don't panic when the phone rings (or you may, but at least you know you have the documents in order).

1. Organize your emergency folder.

   If the first responders are called, they will first ask you for a current list of medications. It is vital that you have up-to-date information in case of emergency. I would still keep the list of medications in a hanging file folder like the rest, but additionally, save a couple of sets of copies in ready-to-go manila envelopes. Don't expect this information to come home from the hospital. If you hand off your list to a doctor, have a copy at home. Don't give the master to the EMTs. For any emergency, you can grab the envelope with the pre-made copies and go. Don't rely on having the list in your phone either because EMTS don't want to bumble around with the list on technology that requires a password every ten seconds.

2. Medical

   Have these ready in a folder: records, health insurance, bills, receipts, past due bills, paid bills, diagnoses letters.

3. Personal

   Birth certificate, will, advanced directive, POLST, power of attorney, marriage certificate, divorce decree, passport, driver's license or id card, social security card, Medicaid card, insurance card, and any other personal document of this nature.

Talking to your parents in advance can get the wheels turning. I know it can be difficult to start these conversations. You might try relating the situation to someone they know. For example, "Mom, do you remember when June was admitted to the hospital, and Frank did not have a clue about what medication she was taking and why? I would hate to have that happen to either of you. I think it would be a good idea to get all of your current medications on a list. How do you feel about that?"

If possible, go to the hospital where you know your doctors have privileges. Privilege is a term used by healthcare facilities to identify physicians who are approved to provide patient services within their facilities. Once you arrive, you may have to wait for extended periods of time, depending upon what is happening. You will be asked to complete heaps of paperwork. New paperwork you need to fill out; this is hard on people. I can tell you that after going to the ER with my mom on an average of twice a month for years, you become numb to the papers. All I could think about was, please help my mom. She is suffering; please don't throw caution to the wind. Make sure you understand what is happening.

When you don't have unlimited resources to just pay extra or above for your parents, it is key you are darn organized and careful with all insurance documents. You need to have a general understanding of the insurance coverage. Is it private pay, Medicare, Medicaid, or something else? There can be benefits available for veterans and other state and county programs that may offer caregiver support. When working with families, I always ask if they have a long-term care policy. These policies may have been written years earlier. Calling the company and reviewing the coverage and specific qualifying factors will determine how to utilize the benefits best.

The Medscape survey from 2016 found that the average time spent with a physician is between 13 and 16 minutes. This is not enough time to understand what is going on with mom and dad. There are so many more questions. When you are receiving information for the first time, often you don't think of the questions you want to ask until later. Then what do you do? The Devoted Daughter provides you with a detailed checklist of questions to ask during a doctor's visit.

We looked for my dad's Medicare card for two years. It was red-tape nonsense. Finally, my brother got fed up and said he was going to pay for his medical expenses out of pocket. We spent countless hours in search of that card. When I finally found it, it was in a place I never would have looked for it. I would also suggest keeping some extra supplies such as folders, files, pens, label maker, etc. nearby so if you need to whip up another folder quickly, it's accessible and will keep everything organized as time goes.

I have witnessed so many cases where a patient was treated in a certain way because of a Medicare billing rule or something equally ridiculous. Why in the world does it make sense to have someone go to the ER for treatment when all they needed was a simple test?

Putting yourself in the shoes of the emergency room staff is the next piece to having a less stressful more orderly emergency situation with a parent. People are walking through the door for random complaints and urgent needs. They work in a very reactive environment and typically don't see the patients for long. If you can establish that human connection with someone working in the ER, you are much more likely to not only get better care but have a better experience.

Did you know that someone can be sent up to a hospital room but not be admitted to the hospital? They could be moved from the ER to the hospital floor for observation only. Admission can be a significant detail that, if overlooked, could end up costing thousands of dollars in unpaid services. The patients whose needs are the highest are treated first. You could even be in the middle of being seen by a doctor, and someone comes in bleeding from the head and all of the sudden you are back in line. Waiting in line at the emergency room is very frustrating; you are there because you have your emergency but others have more pressing situations medically. You are also under stress, so not knowing what is going to happen next can add to your overall anxiety. Stay calm and find someone you can continue to speak to for any updates. I would try to find a nurse working the desk or someone who seemed approachable, to try to establish rapport as quickly as possible.

Here are actions that you can take to start organizing all the other paperwork and documents for your parents, so you feel prepared in case of an emergency. (You don't have to do this in one weekend!)

1. Sort through paperwork and bills

   If you haven't seen your parents for a while, it can take time to find and sort through all the paperwork and bills. Even if you were there yesterday, it could still take time. For your sake and for your parents', try going through one room at a time collecting documents and papers that seem essential. Once you think you're done, you'll likely open another drawer of crucial documents haphazardly shoved away, but try and at least get the bulk of the information. You may need to take the documents home or sort them somewhere out of sight. Digging through things and sorting can make people anxious and raise questions. It can also make your parents feel inadequate, or like you are taking over. If there is one thing I learned from doing Senior Care for the last eleven years, it was to leave people with their dignity. I know well-meaning families, who with limited time and resources take charge to accomplish the task, leaving their parents feeling defeated, sad, angry, you-name-it, the emotions run the gambit. Imagine someone you love more than anything taking over your life with no consideration of your feelings. Making assumptions is a bad idea. Having a conversation and gaining agreement before you take action can save you a lot of hard feelings.

2. Categorize and purge

   Once you have about all the materials you can find together, start laying the items into categories. Get a large space where you can spread out for this, and use whatever system works for you; boxes you can label with a sharpie, post-it note piles, or even write each category on a scrap piece of paper and lay the papers on top of the pile. Close the windows so a draft doesn't blow all your work away, and be mindful of pets that may jump on the piles while you are gone! Whatever works for you, start putting similar items together.

Suggestions for sorting categories:

- Auto—car titles, service and repair receipts, loan information, insurance records, etc.
- Career—education records, paystubs, etc.
- Emergency—copies of necessary documents, personal information sheet, insurances, etc. If you don't have copies made already, make the pile and a mental note to come back later.
- Financial—bank statements, loan information, closed accounts, credit card information, credit reports, mortgage information, etc.
- Taxes—a separate pile for previous years and the current year. The current year would include donations, expenses, paystubs, anything that you'll need to file.

If there are multiple years' worth of documents, you may want to make duplicate categories by year. Additionally, purge through anything that you're sure you won't need. Yes, some things are worth keeping, but chances are there's plenty you can recycle as well. If you're nervous about throwing paperwork away such as expired insurances, you may want to put documents that are questionable in a separate pile. Typically, old receipts and records for stuff you no longer own don't need to stick around.

It's essential you chose a designated area for all your paperwork, so items don't end up getting lost all over again. What you use to contain your papers is entirely up to your preference. Fortunately, now there are many more attractive options than a heavy steel filing cabinet, but if that's what you prefer, use one!

If you or your older adult is not in a permanent home or are planning on moving soon, there are plastic filing tubs with handles that are easy to move. If you're staying put, there are attractive furniture options available, or more box-like choices you can pop in a closet or a cabinet.

If you're running a household with multiple children, a partner, yourself, and your parents, I would recommend a larger container that you could separate your family's on one side and your parents on the other. If your parents are more medically complex, chances are you'll also want a larger container. Do your best to eyeball your current stacks to figure out what size you need before buying anything. If there are tons of necessary paperwork in front of you after you've done a thorough purge, it may be best to purchase several smaller containers for each label.

I recommend good old- fashioned file folders and a label maker to start organizing; I prefer to organize documents alphabetically into categories and subcategories. Your system may be different from mine, but overall, this is a relatively straightforward way to proceed.

Once all your parents' files and materials are labeled and organized, you can put them in a permanent, well-kept spot. Since there are so many essential documents, be careful where the documents are stored. Don't put them in a space that is damp and can be mildewed. The most important documents should be scanned and backed up with technology so you have them on paper and electronically, just in case something happens.

~~~~

Amid all this organizing, at Christmas time, I was able to pause and reminisce with my mom. I was not just able to spend time with her, but I was able to help her re-live the feeling she
~~~~

had as a talented painter and artist. Back then she attended a ceramics class every Wednesday night. It started out as a way to carve out time with her friends, but it developed into a passion project. She was blind now, so she couldn't paint anymore or see her art work, but as she touched the pieces, she reminisced about each unique piece of décor. One of her most proud accomplishments was a nativity scene. She painted every detail and each figurine was bejeweled with dazzling detail. The collection was displayed year round in a curio cabinet in our living room. I placed each of the figurines in her hands and we talked about each one and where she wanted to place it on her mantel. I sensed she was exhausted, so I wanted to capture each and every minute where she could find joy and happiness. Friends and family would be visiting, and I knew she would want her home to be festive and welcoming. The last touch was to hang the wreath on the door and decorate her planter boxes on the front porch.

There is so much to do when taking care of a parent, and striking that balance of being a daughter and a caregiver is complicated. Preparation for emergencies, or when they pass is the responsible action to take, but so is carving out time to be with them and remember who they were and what they brought to your life and this planet; it is necessary for your healing process.

CHAPTER TEN

BRINGING IN HOSPICE

My mom was in physical dire failure. She was terminally ill, now on dialysis three times a week, but the fluid was building and stretching out the skin on her legs so tight, it would burst and ooze. She was suffering from stomach pain, and chronic diarrhea was increasing by the day. It was affecting her ability to eat, and was in turn causing other problems. Even with me owning an in-home care business, I was so wrapped up with being the devoted daughter, I could have paid more attention to health and safety, regardless of whether my mom didn't want someone peeping over her shoulder all the time or not. There is a balance that needs to be factored in when dealing with the emotional rollercoaster of being in charge of your parent. I was also not fully facing that my mom's death was coming. She had been in the fight so long, and I had been there right alongside her.

When you are caring for someone who is ill, you forget that they're are dealing with pain 24 hours a day. You will need to have more compassion, and as a daughter, I wish I had done more in that role than as a worker bee. Someone else could have been doing laundry and going to the grocery store and Fred Meyer to get prescriptions, which would have given me more time to spend with my mom in the last days as her daughter. Again, as someone who doesn't like to sit still very long, I empathize if you are uncomfortable with that level of intimacy. I wanted to just push through and fix it, which did keep her alive longer. Yet at the end of the day, more emphasis could have been put on quality time. Creating special memories when someone is terminally ill is priceless, if it is only just thirty minutes. I also could not help but hope that if we could enjoy these moments, somehow all the other health concerns could go away for a little while. My sister in law, Sarah, was perfect for the intimacy piece, listening to her feelings all the time. If you can't be in that space, find the family member or friend who can provide that to your suffering parent.

At The Devoted Daughter, we put emphasis on the Circles of Care, and I have stressed many times through the preceding chapters that you need to think about the people your family interacts with daily, weekly, and monthly who can be of help to you and your parent. The reason I say family is, like it or not, you are in this together. If you are taking time away from your family to help your parents, how will that impact your life and the lives of your children? I have also implored you to examine the people on the outside of the circle such as are professionals, service companies, people in the community, possibly a bank teller or a grocery store clerk. Many of these types of people have gotten to know your parent over the years and may want to lend a hand with driving or simple socialization when your parent is lonely.

As you approach the center of the circle, you are now identifying people you would call in the middle of the night in case of emergency. It is important to think through who can and who is willing to help in these different circumstances. In my professional experience, I have seen many families who make assumptions that someone is closer to the center of the circle than they should be or are willing to be. Talking about this in advance will clear up some of those misconceptions before it's too late.

~~~~

We started another cycle of going in and out of the hospital, and the nephrologist recommended we see a physician who might have some ideas on how to control her stomach pain. I called and got the first available appointment. It was three weeks out, but maybe this would help. I should have been contacting hospice by now, but I had no idea how helpful and effective they could be. I guess I had to have one more horrendous experience with my mom before I went down on my knees and accepted that I could no longer do everything myself.

On the day of the appointment, I arrived at my mom's house early to help her get ready to go. That was a long process. Getting in the shower, getting dressed, and having scheduled rest breaks in between took at least an hour and a half. I did not want to rush her; she had enough on her plate, so we tried to take as much time as she needed. She did not like to be cold, so I had a space heater in the bathroom. It was a walk-in shower with grab bars. This made it easy for her to sit down in the shower chair and use the hand-held shower wand. She had already lost so much, so anything she could do for herself was a bonus.

Easy shower tips

Hand-held shower wand—These are great and easy to install, but you must buy the brand that fits with your shower head. Unscrew your shower head and screw in the fixture.

If you have a tub, some benches fit over the tub, allowing the person to sit down and slide into the shower. Using the bench in combination with a hand-held shower head could work fabulously.

Remove all tripping hazards in the bathroom. Many of these tips may seem like common sense, but lots of seniors have
~~~~

bathmats and rubber mats in the bathtubs. These can get tangled up and cause a fall. Most falls happen in and around the bathroom.

Warm up towels in the dryer to put on their shoulders and one in their lap while they are showering in the chair. I also offered her warm towels to dry off. You may go through a boatload of towels, but your parent could shower more independently and comfortably this way.

If someone is resistant to showering, break down the process. Start with soaking his or her feet in warm water at first. Maybe later in the day, you could suggest that the doctor recommended that some cream should be applied to the back so you could get clean clothing on the top half of the body. These steps may take a couple days to accomplish, but I have found that breaking it up into baby steps can help.

~~~~

It was mid-February and my mom was hanging on by a thread. We had searched high and low for anyone and anything that could help stabilize her body. Deep down, I knew we were in trouble and running out of options. *Was there a solution? Could she possibly recover?* I did not know, but I was going to try as long as she wanted to search for answers. I would go to the doctor with my mom, and we would see people who were very overweight going about their business with minimal effort. They were not in any way hindered, except for the weight, and my mom was so angry. Why is it that some people can get away with making choices against medical advice, while others suffer as their bodies break down? My mom would say, "Why me? I love my kids and my life; I want to live!" One of my mom's friends spent all her time in the sun in Maui, smoking cigarettes, walking on the beach
~~~~

and reading. I saw her five years ago, and she was in her nineties at that time. She was a great person and was able to make those choices against medical advice and defy the odds. For most of us, it does not work that way. It does not seem fair, but we will never know the answers to those questions. I am saddened that my mom will never see her grandchildren grow up. They will not have the joy of knowing their grandmother, as my brothers and I knew our grandparents. I remember saying to her, "Your mind wants to go shopping, but your body is breaking down." I just prayed for peace and for the pain to subside.

I took matters in my hands one more time in managing her care, and I guess it was a blessing it got completely messed up because it led me to reach out to hospice. I had the name of the clinic she had an appointment with and printed it off the internet with the address information. We arrived about 15 minutes early and I pulled up to the front door. I told my mom I was going to run in and grab a wheelchair so we did not have to fool around with the walker. When I walked into the lobby and looked for the suite number, the physician was not listed in the directory. I went back to the car and called the doctor's office. They were no longer at that address. The new location was across town and it was 1:30 PM. They would not have time to see my mom today. My mom was so hopeful that this doctor would be able to help her. I had to walk away from the car, I was so upset. I felt like a complete loser. How could I have screwed this up? This could be her last shot. I was crying so hard, I knew I had to pull myself together. The only saving grace was my mom could not see the tears streaming down my face. I went back to the car and explained what had happened. She could not understand how the address could be wrong and I told her they had not updated it with the listing company. *Why didn't they tell us?* I don't think they knew. I assured my mom that we would go home and call them again and get back on the books. She was so upset; now we were both crying. It is so awful to be grasping at straws.

I shouldn't have trusted the internet for an appointment this important, but I was stretched too thin to think logically. Someone should have been there helping me, and may have had the foresight to double check the address.

When we got home, I called the doctor's office and begged them for another appointment. They did not have anything for two more weeks, but I said we would take it. The following weekend, we found ourselves back in the hospital. Going to the ER on the weekend is a nightmare. When we got home, I called her primary care physician to speak to him about hospice services. I knew we were out of options with her physical body.

You can only fix so many parts. I was not thinking of it in terms of my mom was going to die. I was looking for more support in-home to help with comfort measures. We needed help to stop the cycle of the emergency room every other day. Some people improve with hospice and are discharged. Her primary care doctor was not on-call, but the person I spoke to was familiar with my mom's case and thought this would be a good idea. Now, I needed to talk to my brothers and my mom to see how they felt. For many people, the word hospice is a death sentence. Typically, you need a referral from your primary care doctor to initiate services if Medicare is paying. Hospice services are intended to offer comfort measures and are not there to extend life. That means if you plan to have open heart surgery, you cannot be on hospice. In the Circles of Care, hospice is part of education, people, and products and services. It crosses three platforms, and The Devoted Daughter covers a lot of questions and tells you many of the ins and outs of hospice you wouldn't know from general inquiry.

I, like many people, waited too long to initiate services with hospice. At The Devoted Daughter, we help you see the benefits of hospice. No one tells you the ins and outs of hospice until someone is almost dead. When you are dealing with healthcare in general, you will likely get a pat on the back and a brochure. Hospice is a gift to offer support to people at home, and it should not be something the evokes fear, but rather a decision to provide more comfort. Both my brothers agreed that hospice could help my mom and keep her out of the emergency room. I was dreading the conversation with my mom, but at this point, I felt strongly that hospice could help. I knew she was going to think we had given up on her. That was not the idea at all! I asked her to agree to a meeting with hospice so we could learn more about what they had to offer. After the meeting, we could decide if this was the right decision for our family. She agreed, although I knew she was scared to death.

The hospice team came to meet with us and talked about their services. I was not aware that they only had an RN visit once a week. *Since my mom was still on dialysis how would that be handled? Is dialysis considered a life-sustaining treatment and therefore she would have to make a choice?* These scenarios present themselves and The Devoted Daughter can offer you the information you need to make educated decisions for your family. I knew the hospice conversation was not going to go over well. The social worker also explained that they have other services such as counseling, volunteer sitter services, and spiritual support. My mom wanted to speak with her doctor about the dialysis before deciding on hospice support. It was agreed that she could continue dialysis as a comfort measure even though she would be admitted to hospice.

On the first day of hospice, the RN and the social worker came to the home to do an intake. It took a couple of hours for them to gather all of the data and formally admit her. One of the things I was not prepared for was the comfort pack. It is a sealed package of medication that is left with every new patient in case of emergency. It was a little scary when they said we might need this if she starts to have anxiety or feels like she can't breathe. I was not sure what they were talking about, so I just let it go. I did not want to think about what was ahead of me; I only had enough bandwidth to deal with what was in front of me at that moment.

They also left a little blue book for the family and encouraged all of us to review the material. When I opened the book, it was all about death. For God's sake, I don't want to read this crap. I am her daughter. I am trying to help my mom stay alive. I don't want to focus on death. I couldn't face the fact that I was going to lose this decades-long fight.

Interestingly enough, my brother and my gram both read the book. They wanted to know and be more prepared for what might be coming down the track. The point is, everyone is different in how they respond and process information. There is no right or wrong. There was no judgment; just a family trying to do the right thing.

At The Devoted Daughter, we have an extensive information bank on hospice tips. Here are some of the tips that I found most helpful when dealing with my mom's situation.

1. Hospice is not a death sentence. People can be admitted and discharged from hospice. If someone decides they want to try a life-saving treatment, they would be released from hospice and go back to their original providers. All the paperwork should be double checked to ensure there is not a lapse in coverage!
2. Hospice has physicians on staff, so once a patient is admitted into the program, he or she relinquishes other providers. Insurance will not cover specialty care if you have entered into an agreement with hospice to provide comfort care.

3. Hospice staff is on call 24 hours a day, but they are not in the patient's home 24 hours a day. They meet with their patients on a scheduled basis. If more care is required, you may need to hire staffing or organize friends and family to support you through this time.

Anytime you have a policy decision, especially when it involves insurance payments, be sure to get that in writing. When my mom was admitted to hospice, they approved dialysis treatments for comfort care purposes. Out-of-policy decisions require approval from the medical team and from Medicare. I had stacks of paperwork for hundreds of doctors' appointments, etc. Thankfully, I had all of them in a file. A couple months after my mom died, the hospital started calling me to collect for the dialysis treatments. I had all my ducks in a row, and I was able to prove that her insurance covered it. In the stress of someone dying or even someone who is ill, paperwork is the last thing you have on your mind, but it is crucial that you stay organized. At The Devoted Daughter, we provide organizational tips on how to keep the stacks of paperwork caught up. It is hard enough to grieve and lose a loved one, let alone to think about paperwork, but it is vitally important that you keep your documents in one place even if they are not organized. I threw papers in a bin so they were safe, and I knew where to find them when I was up to the task of organizing.

My mom continued her dialysis treatments and we continued to hope for the best. Her stomach issues were not getting any better; in fact, they were getting worse. It was so bad that even a sip of water would trigger diarrhea. The nephrologist decided to try a tincture of opium. The side effect of the drug is constipation and we were hopeful it would control diarrhea. It is a potent drug. One afternoon when I was with my mom, I gave her a dose of the opium. She was laying down in bed and I warned her that it was powerful and it could make her dizzy, so she needed to stay down to prevent falling. As I was getting ready to leave, my sister in law was coming over. My mom's manicurist was also planning to stop by. I told my mom that Sarah would be there in ten minutes and that she should not get up. About a half hour later Sarah called and said my mom got out of bed and fell against the door. She warned me that her face looked like she had been in an automobile accident. I thought, *I should never have left her alone.* We called hospice right away and asked the nurse to come over and evaluate her injuries. When I got back there, her face was swollen and red; it looked awful.

The hospice nurse arrived, and she was pretty hard on me. She said that my mom needed 24-hour care and that I was irresponsible in leaving her. A recommendation for 24-hour care came out of the blue with this accident, and I felt bad not knowing this fact. I was trying to honor my mom's wishes and allow her some privacy, but it was clear we needed to get more help. There are times in life when you are so close to something that you can't see clearly. I know now that is what was happening to me. I was so entrenched in the day-to-day care that at times I lost sight of the big picture. Although we had some care in place and friends and family were involved on a daily basis, you can never have enough resources when you are supporting a terminally ill person. Make the time to get help sooner rather than later. Logically, I knew what needed to be done, but I decided to honor my mom and let her have the final say. My mom was resistant, but I told her that it was just not safe for her to be alone all the time. We would start to take turns spending the night from then until she got stronger.

The following week, I called my mom in the morning as usual. She did not answer, so I kept calling and calling. As I was calling, I was getting myself together to get in the car and check in on her. It was unusual for her to not answer the phone after multiple calls. I had this pit in my stomach that something was not right. I lived about 40 minutes away. When I arrived, she was still in bed, but unresponsive. I called hospice immediately and said I needed someone asap. Nurse Nancy called me back and asked me a bunch of questions. She was asking what color her feet were. I was so angry; I just wanted someone to help us. I needed someone there now; it was an emergency. I was there all alone, and I did not know what to do. I called David to let him know, and he said he was on his way. The next call was to my brother, Chris, in Arizona, and I told him, "You have to get here as soon as possible." I was not sure if I was losing her. The phone rang and it was the social worker. I explained what was happening, and she said she would be right over. When the social worker arrived, my mom was moving slightly, but she was drifting in and out of consciousness. I expressed my displeasure with nurse Nancy, but she was already on her way.

The next few days were touch and go. Hospice assigned a new RN to manage my mom's case.

The relationship you develop with the hospice team is critical. I can't imagine how difficult it must be working with terminal patients and struggling families day in and day out. Hospice makes it possible for families to remain together and support one another. We had spent years in and out of hospitals, nursing homes, and assisted living facilities and there is no place like home. I will admit this was one of the hardest times in my life and I know I was not an easy person to deal with at that time. That being said, I was my mom's advocate, I was fighting for her life. I felt like we were in a war zone fighting an unknown battle, knowing we might never get out alive. Finding the balance between what is best for the patient and being realistic about what is medically possible is a puzzle. My mom was too ill to speak for herself, so I felt an overwhelming responsibility to make sure I communicated clearly on her behalf.

My mom's condition had changed, but she was able to get out of bed and spend some time in the family room. She was speaking and using the bathroom with assistance. For the first time, I started to come to grips with the fact that this was the beginning of the end. Until this point, I had a glimmer of hope that something might change. We called a family meeting with hospice to discuss the care plan. My mom had not received any dialysis treatment for over a week. She was unable to get out of bed and go to dialysis. My heart broke for her as we talked to her about discontinuing her dialysis treatment. She sat in the chair looking scared and frail, and trying to process the news that continuing the treatments would not sustain her life. Later that day, I was helping her in the bathroom, and she was sobbing and crying saying, "It's just not fair; I love my kids and I don't want to leave you." I looked up at her and said, "I know, mom. We don't want you to leave; we love you. Your mind wants to jump up and get dressed and go shopping, but your body is broken."

How to prepare for a loved one's death

- Find someone to take the pressure down for you so you can sink into the role of daughter, granddaughter, or niece, so you can experience your loved one's death, not as a taskmaster.
- Figure out what matters. What is impactful on your life and your parent's life in the final days? Time is something you will never get back.
- Spending time with your parents during their last days is a very personal experience, and for each person it is different. Allow your family members the space to grieve and say their goodbyes without judgment.
- Find a way to support one other through the process.

Early one morning as my mom slept, the cat started bouncing off the walls, and I mean literally running into walls. It was as if her animal instincts were trying to tell us something. My brother and his wife were staying with my mom and woke to the ruckus. As my brother approached my mom, she said, "I think today is the day." None of us wanted to acknowledge what was happening, but we knew we were treading on thin ice. I did not want to talk about her dying, and when I arrived, we sat quietly on the bed together. We were alone, and I wanted to do what I could to offer her comfort and support. She was no longer able to get out of bed, and she was taking high doses of medication for pain. Just moving her head slightly caused an immense amount of pain and dizziness. I got her some soda and she took a small sip. One sip caused her to have diarrhea. My first instinct was to get her cleaned up, but she was in so much pain, I could not do anything. She could not move a muscle without screaming out in pain. I thought to myself, *This is ok; once the pain medication kicks in, I will be able to get her cleaned up.* That never happened.

Throughout the morning and into the early afternoon we took turns sitting with my mom in her room. The family gathered in the living room, and at times, things got loud. I remember struggling with the noise, and I knew it was bothering my mom. Everyone was anxious, and that anxiety presents itself in different ways. One by one, we would take turns sitting quietly with my mom, holding her hand to make sure she knew we were there.

By late afternoon, my mom was crying out to call 911, saying she could not breathe. Hospice provides an emergency medication kit for this situation. When I went to get the medication, it was gone! I was frantic, and Chris was distraught, where in the hell was the medicine? I called hospice in a sheer panic asking them what we should do. They asked a couple questions, and then we remembered that we had a strong medication we could use until there was another plan. That bought us some time until we finally located the comfort pack from hospice. I will never forget the feeling of my mom saying she could not breathe. It was god awful.

Once we had her pain stabilized, we continued to administer the medication as needed. Watching her fade away was heart-wrenching. We were all crammed into her room, sitting on the bed; one by one saying our goodbyes and telling her how much we loved her. I have heard people say that you go out as you lived and my mom was a fighter until the minute she took her last breath.

Part of the hospice in-take process guides you through decisions that need to happen down the road. One of those is the funeral home. I remember seeing the paperwork on the funeral home for the first time, and it felt surreal. We had talked about my mom's wishes a million times, so we knew she wanted to be cremated; now it was a matter of selecting a provider. Making that decision in advance made it easier when it was time to make the call. I have to be honest, I wanted to get out of there once she was gone. My gram was not with us and someone needed to tell her. I cannot imagine what it would be like to outlive your daughter and witness how much pain she was in. My gram's brother had died of a massive heart attack in his forties, so she had watched her mom lose a child. She would always say to me, "It's just not natural to lose your child;" she knew how hard it was on her mom, and that she was not the same after that.

David and Chris left to make that dreadful drive to Salem to see Gram. I needed to clear my head and face what had just happened. I walked out to a bright, crisp night and looked up to see the brilliant white of the full moon staring back at me. *What was next?* I was not sure. I could not make sense of anything. In fact, I had been fighting for so long, I couldn't even fathom that it was over. I had been fighting against an inevitability for so long and was entrenched in every detail. I know you are not thinking of yourself right now, but this is the time when you should be thinking of yourself. Be gentle, kind, and take time to process. Pushing forward and keeping busy was my way of coping. There's nothing like putting your head in the sand, but the grief will catch up with you. I was working with a family who was going through the hospice intake process, and I found myself sobbing uncontrollably. I did not know where this was coming from, but my role as a professional was to support the family. I needed to take time to process and heal from my mom's death, and I would encourage you to do the same.

The next morning, I woke up lost and afraid. My entire identity had been wrapped up in caring for my mom and communicating with friends and family about updates. I was paralyzed in indecision about my future. Unsure of what to do next, we decided that her apartment should be cleaned. I wanted to wait a little longer, but it was nearing the end of the month, and rent would be due soon. I knew that it made sense to get this done, and somehow having something to do made us feel like we were still helping my mom. We rushed the whole process and it took years to find some of the belongings we had put in boxes.

I see now that I didn't give myself that time because I was building a business and still taking care of my gram, driving an hour and 20 minutes each way to help her a few days a week. I was filling a void in my life to avoid facing what I was going to do with myself. I could've stopped. I could've hit the pause button, but it was easier to go than stop. When you are used to taking care of somebody all the time and then it just stops, that is part of your identity. Suddenly that part of you is gone. You may be asking yourself if there is anything you can do in advance. The answer is yes. Create a circle of care for yourself. We talk about self-care and caring for the caregiver, but no one talks about the PTSD that happens when you lose a loved one. Caring for your physical well-being and mental health is vital. Days turn into weeks and weeks turn into months and before you know it, you are back at work living your life. As you look at your circle of family and support, set a goal to reach out to at least one person in your circle each week. Start to re-build your social and family connections.

CHAPTER ELEVEN

NOTHING PREPARES YOU FOR DEATH

I missed my mom and so did my gram. We shared that loss and the secure connection of family. The grieving process is different for everyone. I knew my mom wanted to do more for her mom, and if she had been able, she would have done more caregiving, like the trap I had fallen into. In the epicenter of it all, I was caring for my mom and my gram, and instead of being a daughter or a granddaughter in a way that enhanced our relationship and maximized the intimacy, until the very end.

How to celebrate the death after:

For each family, the choice of how to celebrate someone's life is a personal decision. Some people don't even have a preference, but in my mom's case, she was adamant about that until the day she died. She didn't want us to waste any time or money on a service. She didn't believe in it, so why would we do it? Her friends and family members were distraught. They wanted to celebrate her life and lifelong friendships. Making this decision can be heart-wrenching when you are in such an emotional state of mind. The Devoted Daughter outlines many strategies for talking with your parents about these delicate issues.

We knew there needed to be at the very least an announcement of my mom's passing. In honor of her wishes, we sent a letter to her friends and family with a poem in remembrance of her life. I wanted every detail to be something she would be proud of. The notecards were embossed by hand, and the envelopes were sealed with a wax cross. I have memories of writing letters with my mom and sealing them with wax. Sealing that last envelope, tears ran down my cheeks, knowing this would be the final letter. We asked for donations in her name to The American Diabetes Association. This was our way of honoring my mom's wishes and acknowledging the amazing daughter, sister, mother, and friend she was to all who had the pleasure of knowing her. She will take with her the legacy of a family devoted to honoring the person that gave them life.

My mom's ashes sat at the funeral home for months. I knew they needed to be picked up, but I could not get myself to go over there. My brother finally went and picked them up. He called me and said, "Mom's ashes are appropriately boxed with a beautiful pink bow." Pink was her favorite color. My mom's favorite place on the face of the earth was Maui, Hawaii. We decided the best place to celebrate her life would be Maui and her ashes would be scattered in Maalaea Bay. It took us three years to arrange a time when all three of us and our families could be in Maui. We all stayed in the same condos we stayed in as children. The Kihei Canoe Club was next door. We arranged a day to meet on the beach and gather together in celebration of my mom. The ocean was breaking against the shore; it was peaceful and calm. Before getting into the canoes, my niece Sadie read a poem that my great grandma Burnside had written. As she spoke, the tears ran down my cheeks; I was trying to stay strong, but the years of memories came flooding back. There was Hawaiian music in the background and some traditional Hawaiian words of wisdom. We boarded the canoes, each of us wearing orchid leis.

As we paddled out, we began to spread her ashes in the sea while pulling orchids from the leis. The orchids danced across the top of the white caps, drifting away from the canoe. She was finally home.

~~~~

We grew up spending a lot of time with our grandparents. Supporting my gram and spending time with her was not foreign or obligatory in any way. I loved my gram more than I can tell you, but we spent a lot of our time together reminiscing about my mom. It was as if she was still with us, but she wasn't. When someone dies young, the finality is harder to accept than when someone has lived a long life. We created a co-dependent relationship through our grief, but we enjoyed every minute with one another. I looked forward to my gram greeting me at the door. She was always filled with excitement and joy, pinching my cheeks and squeezing me so hard I thought I would pop. My nieces now complain that I do that to them! "No, I don't," I protest, then I caught myself doing it! I threw myself into work, trying to buy myself time to figure out what was next. Since my job was caring for others, I continued filling myself up by giving back to the families we served. What I did not recognize was that I was not everyone else's daughter or granddaughter, and I hadn't even been able to be a daughter or granddaughter in my own family. I had always been a caregiver without boundaries to my family, and learned from my mistakes, so it made sense I would bring those teachings into my business. In the first few years, my in-home care business was all over the map, but I am happy now in retrospect because I was able to work with families firsthand and learn about their real concerns and what was waking them up at night. The information and the experiences were
~~~~

invaluable. When I sold the in-home care company, I was told I was a walking database of information about elder care!

I had clients in Salem near my gram, so I tried to make the most of my drive time by being productive in my business. I realized when I went back to my gram's house, I was driving here every single day and I was not doing it for myself. I was a professional by day, advising families on the importance of boundaries and getting help, but I was not doing that in my own life. My gram kept saying she didn't need my constant care, but naturally, I kept doing everything with her. I finally had the foresight to sit down with my uncle and say, "I want to be the granddaughter, not the caregiver." I knew I had to nip this in the bud before I fell back into the role of caregiver.

I had to break myself from the pattern because I didn't want to lose my role as a granddaughter like I did as a daughter to my mom. I didn't want to be the one giving her baths. I wanted to be her granddaughter. The family was on board with hiring a caregiver, but my gram, not so much. I asked her to give it a try for my uncle and me. I knew this was a big request. She was in an independent living facility. I hired a caregiver named Jen. When Jen came in to help my gram, Gram kept sending her home.

"I don't need you; I am fine today."

Getting her to accept the help was a process. We agreed that there were things Gram could use help with like the laundry and running errands, but every time Jen did the laundry, Gram was right on her tail micromanaging everything. Even though she was mad about the caregivers, she had someone to boss around. It was giving her some of the control back. When she figured out she had wheels, the first thing she did was have them take her back over to the house. Getting back in and seeing what had been done and not been done gave her something to talk about and put her back in the game. She was on the phone with Jerry, the landscaper, giving him hell about her yard. Gram was tough as nails, and she did not want anyone telling her what she could and could not do.

My gram was diagnosed with esophageal cancer. Her doctor was unable to find another case of someone her age with this diagnosis. She was 99 at the time. Gram made the decision not to seek treatment unless it would help to control pain and keep her comfortable. We had hospice come in and meet with the family. This approach was the best support system to manage her pain and establish a relationship with a medical team. Fortunately, my brother who is a physician, and his wife had re-located close to my gram. It was awesome to have more family close by to visit and provide support. We were circling the wagons so the more, the merrier.

One afternoon I stopped in to visit Gram, and the hospice nurse, her caregiver, Jen, and a bath aid from hospice were all there. My gram pulled me aside into another room, and she said, "Never in my life have I had a man help me with a bath."

I told her there was not a man in the house and she insisted that hospice had sent a male bath aid. She was carrying on so loud, everyone heard the conversation. I asked her to sit tight, and I went to investigate. It turned out the woman who she thought was a man had very short hair and was dressed in what could have been men's clothing; I had some insight into her perception of the situation. When you are dealing with someone who is almost 100 years of age, that generation can be judgmental when it comes to gender issues. I suspected this was not the first time this had happened to this individual, as she did not seem alarmed. Perception is 99% of the game, and we were not going to change Gram's mind. My advice on this is not to overreact. If you can handle these types of embarrassing situations with grace, it will benefit everyone in the long run.

Gram passed away in the spring of the following year, two days before her hundredth birthday. Everyone wanted everything wrapped up in fifteen minutes. Then I started spinning. My world felt like it was over; there was no one else in the family to save. The two most influential people in my life were gone forever. I put my head down and started working like crazy, taking on every client I could. I thought I had learned my lesson, but when I had no one, I went back into work full force. I transferred my energy into caring for a business and other people. I don't regret the eight years that transpired; I met people who had better boundaries with their parents and were able to be the son or daughter that I was incapable of with my family, and I could bring that education to others through The Devoted Daughter.

With my mom, my gram, and my dad, I was experiencing the aftermath that one wouldn't see in a caregiving profession. When a parent or family member dies, it is hardly over. Emotions run wild. You are trying to think logically, but everything is a blur. The experience of death is so different for everyone. In fact, the loss of my mom, Gram, and dad were so uniquely as personal as was my relationship with each of them while they were alive. I was doing most of the caregiving work with my mom so I was missing out on the gift of being a daughter. I was raw from the natural emotions of loss and grief, but also the personal fight I had engaged in as a caregiver through all her appointments, and daily hour-by-hour safety and health issues. With Gram, we had more help, so I could be in the natural granddaughter role. With my dad, I was on the outside.

I knew with my gram that I wanted to organize differently than I did with my mom and create a system to how we went through her personal items. With my mom, I made the mistake of trying to do too much too soon. I am not sure what went where. We were making decisions fast and furiously, and putting my mom's personal belongings aside that we would want to go through later. Many of those things were placed in storage or divided between the three of us to sort through at another time. When several people are packing and making decisions, random items get thrown in boxes. Even if the boxes are labeled, something ultimately gets put in a box that is not marked with that item, and you hunt for it for years. I realize that not everyone has the luxury of paying for storage, but maybe you could carve out space in your home or a friend's house until you can sort through the personal items of your past beloved with a clear head. Organization aside, you are owed the opportunity to reminisce and grieve in your own time. There are also professional organizations that will come in and liquidate property and do all the heavy lifting. Retaining the role of daughter, son, or granddaughter also applies to post mortem.

Caregiving is not a linear experience. Your needs change as time passes. The Devoted Daughter Circles of Care houses data that intersects at various times. For example, when someone passes away, there are timely tasks that need to be addressed, but there are also tasks that can be done over time. The family and people circle may be front and center. It could be intersecting with the education and technology circles to help you accomplish your most immediate needs. There are no rules when it comes to processing the death of someone you love. The Circles of Care will help you plan your next steps and bring clarity during a time of despair.

What should be done immediately post-mortem

- Get rid of the super powerful drugs. Unsavory people will discover there has been a death of someone sick or elderly, and they know all those drugs are accessible in a home. The home becomes a target for a break-in.
- Donate durable medical equipment right away that people could use. You don't need to store them or keep

them. They are not personal or emotional. We had bags of wipes, diapers, walkers, wheelchairs, grabbers, canes, you name it, we had it, and we definitely no longer needed any of it, but someone else absolutely did.

- Food and perishables will spoil, so get them into the hands of people who can use them.
- Get a change of address in right away.

What you can wait on

- Family pictures and items about the past. You don't want to stow them away deep in a storage unit like we did, when you could have some fun down the road reminiscing. Chris, David, and I went through the storage unit at least five years after my mom died and we found items we had never seen before. That could have been part of the grieving process more immediately, but they had been buried in the quick exit out of the apartment.

What you can donate

- Furniture can be quickly cleared out. You can have an estate sale once personal items are taken out. There are companies you can hire to do this, which creates income and takes the challenge out of mucking out the house.
- Books, which are heavy. We had sets of Encyclopedias and my dad's collections of medical books. We were hauling those around, thinking that the grandkids would look at these someday; it is highly unlikely, since textbooks are even obsolete in the schools.
- Kitchen items, which are often a bunch of rusted junk, were packed away and stored. A colander that had been painted white—have some lead in your food! An excellent example of people just packing everything. Take that

> time to sort all those items out. There are old metal pans no one wants to use.

You can't save everything, so pick the items that are the most special. If there are items you can't decide on, put those aside for a while. You have your own home and you don't need it filled with your parents' stuff. My mom has been gone for eleven years and just last Christmas, I finally organized her Christmas decorations. It was very personal, so it took me a long time to do the sorting. This is the perfect example of that one area that needs to wait; put it aside until you are emotionally ready to tackle it.

Why do we place so much meaning on our personal belongings? It is just stuff. I've struggled to let go of this stuff for years but there are a few treasures I will keep (family photos, letters, and items that can be passed on to future generations). There are boxes of slides we plan to have digitized so we can enjoy them. I remember sitting in my gram's living room with the slide projector sitting on a tv tray projecting family time images on the screen. Photos are so readily available on our phones that we miss out sitting down together. I wanted to preserve these memories for my nieces so I finally resolved that I would sort through the boxes piled in my storage unit and offer them to family one last time. If no one accepts the items, they will be donated. I found a donation site in my neighborhood that is staffed by volunteers and all the proceeds go to help cancer patients in our community. It feels right knowing that any funds raised will go directly back to people who need the help now. My mom volunteered for years at a local thrift store. They raised money for children to have proper healthcare, including dental work. I know she would be pleased with my decision to help others. Find a cause that speaks to you and follows your heart.

CHAPTER TWELVE

YOUR NEW CAREGIVING PATH

People called my in-home care agency for one of two reasons; either the care need was urgent, or they were looking for more information on how they could help their parents. In either case, I was responding to a demand based on a particular service offering. I created The Devoted Daughter to focus on and answer the most comprehensive questions that came to me during my eleven years in elder care, and to also help you to find the support you need so you can retain the role of son or daughter. Whether it is through one-on-one support or a Facebook group, in person workshops, or self-study at The Devoted Daughter, I can simplify the overwhelming process of elder care and get you to the resource you are looking for as quickly as possible. Weeding through websites and hearing a million different recommendations from well-intended friends who know they have the answer to your prayers is not the way to go.

A few years ago, I met a lovely woman named Ann who was looking for help for her mother. Ann had been through a lot in recent years. Her husband had been diagnosed with cancer, and her mother had dementia and needed to be moved from her home.

Ann's Story

"I was struggling to spend time with my family and find the best solution for my mother. Kelli helped me find fantastic caregivers who bonded with my mom and allowed me to spend some quality time with my husband and children. Spending time with my family was the goal, but little did I know how important this would become. Kelli's agency had been caring for my mother for about a year. One morning I called Kelli on her cell.

"'Ann, are you ok?' she asked.

"'I have some news, I am going to need more help,' I replied.

"'Sure. How can I help?' Kelli responded.

"'I lost my husband Jon last week, and I have been diagnosed with terminal cancer.'

"Kelli was as stunned as I was. Jon and I were both in the prime of our lives with two adult children. We had worked hard to build a life for our kids, and now these kids have lost their dad, and who knows how long I would live? Despite this horrible news, I was relatively calm. I told Kelli my son would be coming home to stay with me during treatment, but he would also be working, and I did not want my health to interfere with his life. Kelli met with us the following day. She was surprised to see how frail and weak I had become, but my spirit remained strong."

I cared for Ann until her passing over the next four months.

Ann's mom was unable to comprehend that her daughter had passed away. Her mom was living with dementia. I had so much experience to impart for the family in this area. Ann's children were paralyzed with grief and since Ann had been the primary caregiver for her mother, someone would need to take over that role. Instead of hiring me, a close family friend stepped in to direct Ann's mother's care. What happened from there was the classic example of a close-knit family suddenly torn apart by cancer.

Ann's mother became a by-product of the circumstances. She was moved from her home within the month. The caregivers she had known were also removed. The family friend insisted that this is how she dealt with her parents and this would be best for Ann's mom. Although these actions were well intended, and someone needed to take charge, it was heartbreaking to watch the unraveling of all the care Ann had put in place for her mom. I knew in my heart this is not what Ann would have wanted for her mother, but the decisions were out of my hand; I was a paid professional, not a family member. These scenarios bring me to speak openly about The Devoted Daughter and explain that this scenario could have been avoided if a documented roadmap had been created by Ann and her mom that her son could have followed post mortem, rather than leave it in the hands of a family friend. The talk about what to do after death could have been facilitated.

~~~~

As there continues to be an imbalance in direct care, I find it more important than ever that I serve more people with my knowledge through The Devoted Daughter. I find myself asking the question, *How can I make a difference in more lives and support people struggling to find solutions while in the midst of the emotional rollercoaster of caring for their aging parents?*

Again, I can't say enough that the process is not linear when finding solutions for people as they age. For example, someone can have a medical event that throws the entire family off balance, and then they get better and things are back to normal for a little while. Also, each individual situation is unique depending on his or her health issues and personality.
~~~~

While I had my in-home care company, I received a call from Janet asking me if we could work with folks who had feeding tubes. That was a red flag because there are rules and regulations around this type of care.

Janet's Story

"Kelli met with me and I explained to her that my Aunt Pam had left a memory care facility against medical advice. The mailman found her on her kitchen floor four months earlier. We had no idea that the house was in such a horrible state with papers, trash, old food, medications, and valuables buried in piles around the house. Aunt Pam also was living with dementia along with her other medical conditions. Kelli told us the first thing we needed to do was put together a plan with the rest of the family. We were a bit shocked to learn the intensity of what was needed for Aunt Pam. Ten caregivers were hired; that is right, count them, ten. And they would all need to be supervised by an RN. Kelli coordinated the efforts with home health so Aunt Pam would have medical coverage 24 hours a day. Fortunately, Aunt Pam was able to afford the care. I know that most people would not be able to afford this level of care. I am so happy, though, that Kelli pushed our family to plan for the future before something catastrophic happened."

I have said this a number of times, but the number-one mistake people make is waiting too long to get help. Identify options in your state, county, and even Veteran's benefits that might pay for care.

There is a second part of the story with Pam that is the epitome of the value of good care. Pam was a woman who was very wealthy, traveled all over the world, and had her PhD. One of the caregivers was in her early twenties and loved Pam like she was her own grandmother. The two of them found common ground. A personal connection is not something you can predict, but I am glad her family was open to accepting help from a person who was from a different social status. One day, I arrived to find the caregiver and Pam ballroom dancing in the living room. What a sight for sore eyes. That moment was pure joy for Pam and the caregiver. They were giggling and prancing around the living room. To this day, thinking of that warms my heart, and moments just like these are why I founded The Devoted Daughter. Amid all the upheaval financially, logistically, and emotionally of aging, people can find joy in their lives even as their health is declining because of age. Pam would have never seen that kind of pleasure in a memory care unit. The memories of her late husband and their home surrounded her. We were able to care for Pam in her own home and keep her safe by organizing and putting a plan together. Without the efforts of the entire team, Pam would not have been able to live at home and would have lived out her days in a memory care setting. She would not pass away amid stress and her family would not be taxed.

~~~~

We also need to understand that our parents are losing their independence and they will push back and fight to keep what they have. My gram fought tooth and nail to stay in her home. She thought she was fine living alone. She had great neighbors, but it is not the responsibility of a neighbor to be your caregiver. It was not until she suffered mobility problems that she agreed it was no longer safe to stay at home.

One scenario that is common in older adults who have been married for years is they support one another in their weakness. One person drives, the other one cooks; one person talks on the phone, the other one reads the mail. One link goes missing and suddenly, your parents need more help to remain independent.
~~~~

It is hard to think about your parents aging. Aging can be gradual, with things slowing down over time, or an unexpected event or illness can hit your family like a Mack truck. Even if your parents are not facing an immediate change in status, you can't stop father time. Start the conversation with your parents and your siblings now. Learn from one another, reflect on childhood memories, and determine next steps. You don't have to have a plan from beginning to end, but at least put one foot in front of the other so you don't have any regrets. I made a promise to my mom that I would never let her go back to a skilled nursing home again no matter what. The promise was fulfilled, but I would not recommend putting that kind of pressure or guilt on your shoulders. You can't predict the future, and someone's health can force your hand to make an unpopular decision. My gram's dad made her promise to never put her mom in a home. That was the way they referred to skilled nursing at the time. Once her dad passed away, her mom's dementia progressed, and she was not safe at home alone. My gram was forced to make the unpopular decision to put her in a home. She agonized over this until the day her mom passed away.

I know that not every family has the resources to go it alone, so start planning to get help. Review your Circles of Care at least twice a year and remember to include tasks that can be automated, like grocery shopping with a delivery service. Resources and needs change over time so stay on top of who is doing what.

Aging parents and their specific care needs are an inevitability that many people are not facing, then it lands on their plate in a landslide or a whirlwind. All they know is other people who have been there. What if those people giving advice also don't have a good game plan or organization? Now, it's the blind leading the blind, and you have no idea the breadth and the weight of this kind of responsibility, the support that is needed to survive it. People live in all parts of the US, and for that matter, the world.

Technology makes our global economy a reality, but when it comes to your parent's care, technology doesn't solve it all.

There are times in life when you can't see the forest through the trees. You are so close to someone or something that a solution seems utterly impossible. Pick your battles and the best time to have a conversation. Evaluate hot buttons so you can anticipate objections. For example, mom might think she has plenty of money to afford assisted living in her town. Most seniors who have been living in their own homes for many years are out of touch with the rising cost of living. You might start by giving her the real cost of living, moving, etc. By offering the facts and not challenging her, you might be able to have a discussion rather than an argument. The Devoted Daughter offers you suggestions on how to approach your family in these challenging situations. Maybe she does have the funds, but this is something you need to know to make plans for the future.

How can we help? For more ideas on how you can work with my team, check out www.thedevoteddaughter.com. Our mission is to help you weed through the volumes of information and point you in the right direction as quickly and painlessly as possible. Care is a continual process, and it does not have to be a headache. You don't have to go it alone. Getting help can bring you back to the role of daughter or son, and in my opinion, that is invaluable. My biggest regret was spending my time with my mom as a caregiver instead of as a daughter. I am honored that I was given the opportunity to serve over a thousand families in the last eleven years through my in-home care business. I have seen people go from complete overwhelm to engaging with their parents. Having more help and support can give you back the relationship with your parents you may have thought was lost forever.

Nothing can be more valuable than that peace of mind.

About the Author

Kelli is a native Oregonian who has dedicated the last twenty years of her life both personally and professionally to senior care. Kelli's mom was diagnosed with Diabetes many years ago, and she suffered multiple complications ranging from blindness to kidney failure. If that was not enough, she also battled breast and pancreatic cancer. It was during that time that Kelli realized they were not the only family struggling to find solutions for care. That realization led her to own and operate a nationally recognized in-home care company. Over the next decade, Kelli served hundreds of families helping them to navigate the ins and outs of caring for an aging family member. Being on the other side of the fence gave Kelli a unique perspective on senior care. You will find those hidden gems in the book.

But something was missing! Kelli knew there was more to help families than in-home care. The Devoted Daughter was born — a comprehensive resource for family caregivers. To learn more about her services you can visit thedevoteddaughter.com. Kelli's social media links are displayed on her website as well.

Made in the USA
Monee, IL
08 November 2026

67378663R00085